Ella the Dog

written by

Dargie Arwood

and

Alex, Alexis, Alexis, Andrew, Autumn, D'Andre, Erika, Ethan, George, Joshua, Katy, Mark, and Zachary

illustrated by

Jessica Cappell and Dargie Arwood

Published by Arc of Anderson County Publishing
109 Dewey Road
Oak Ridge, Tennessee 37830

First printing, May 2018
Printed in the United States of America

Library of Congress Cataloging in Publication Data
Arwood, Dargie, 1958 -
Ella the Dog
Dargie Arwood

ISBN: 978-0-692-10586-3
1. Service Dogs 2. DisAbilities 3. fostering/adoption dogs 4. kindness

Library of Congress Control Number: 2018940681

Design & Layout   Barbara M Lee

Red Horseshoe
Books™
Powell, Tennessee

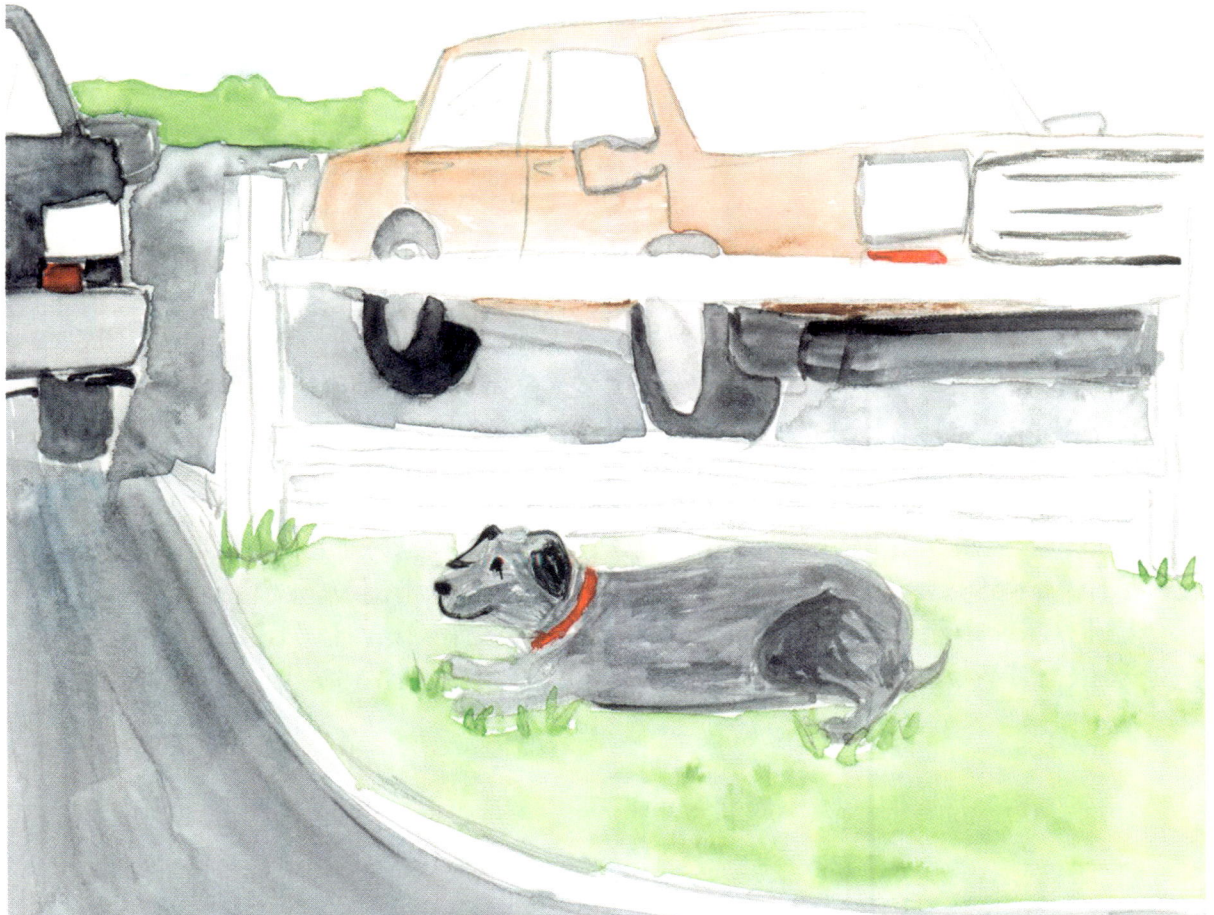

Ella was tired, hungry, and frightened as she walked slowly along the fence line. Cars were moving all around her and she didn't know where to go to be safe.

She spotted some cars that were sitting still and decided to hide by them. It was getting chilly on this busy Friday night and Ella's stomach rumbled as she sniffed the wonderful aroma coming from the people passing by carrying funnel cakes, cinnamon bread, and popcorn. She could hear screaming from the roller coasters and a man welcoming people as they rode by on the trolley.

Suddenly, there was a man standing in front of Ella. She didn't know what to do. She wanted to run, but she was afraid to go back outside the fence where the cars were moving. Ella stood very still and waited to see if the man was going to hurt her. He had a kind voice and she was so glad to see him kneel down and offer her his hand. This lovely black dog with a breastplate shaped white patch in front needed a friend.

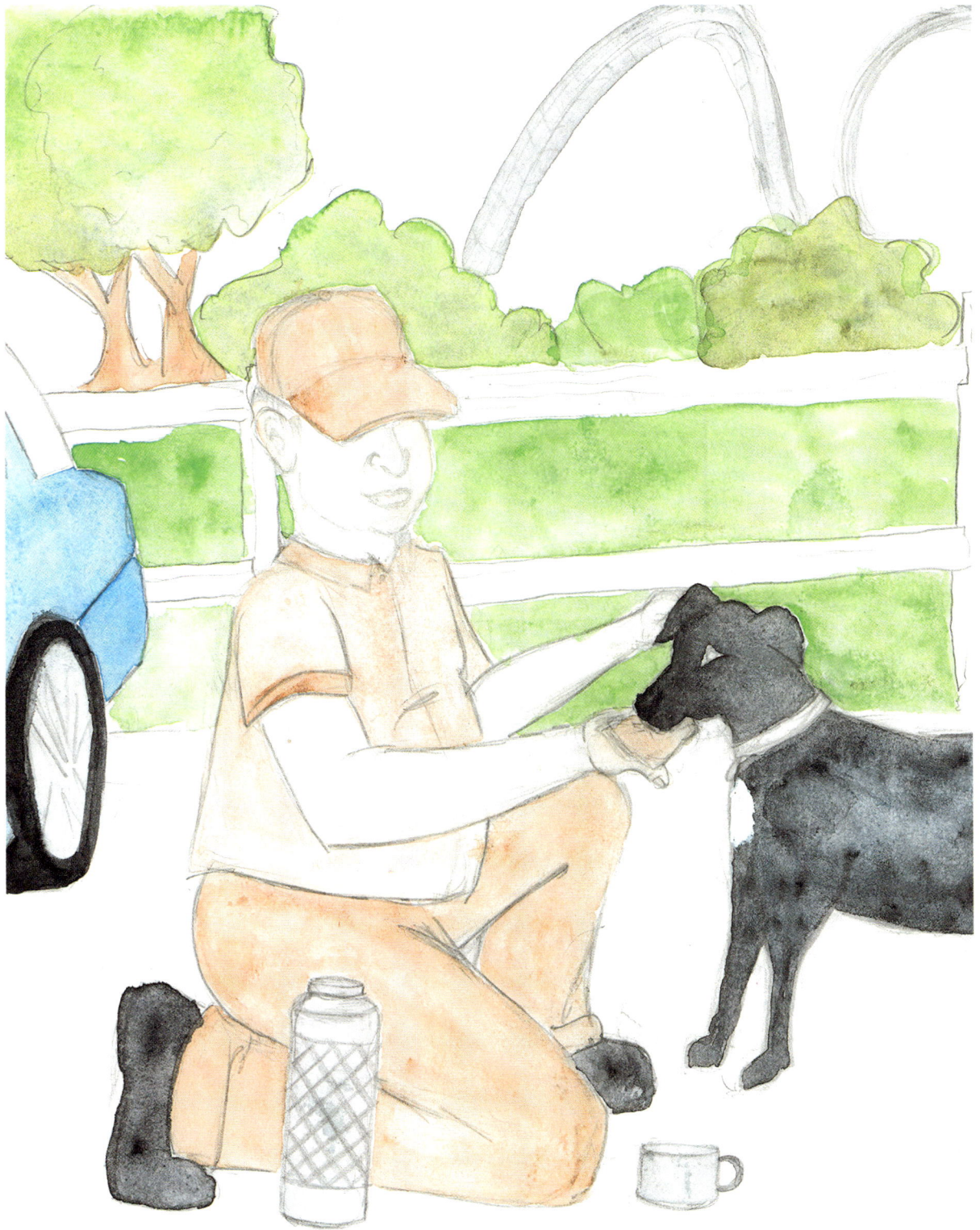

Bill spoke softly to Ella, "Hi, little one, I'm Bill. You look hungry." He offered her the peanut butter sandwich that was in his lunch bag. Ella gobbled up the sandwich then wished she had some water. Bill loved dogs, so he knew that Ella must be thirsty. He used his thermos cup to offer Ella water from a bottle. She drank quickly and waited for more. She looked at Bill with tired eyes after she drank her fill.

Bill cautiously put his hand down again for Ella to sniff. He waited to pet her until she seemed comfortable with him. "Sweet girl, let me look at your tags. Okay, you are Ella from Florida. How did you travel all the way from Florida to Dollywood?

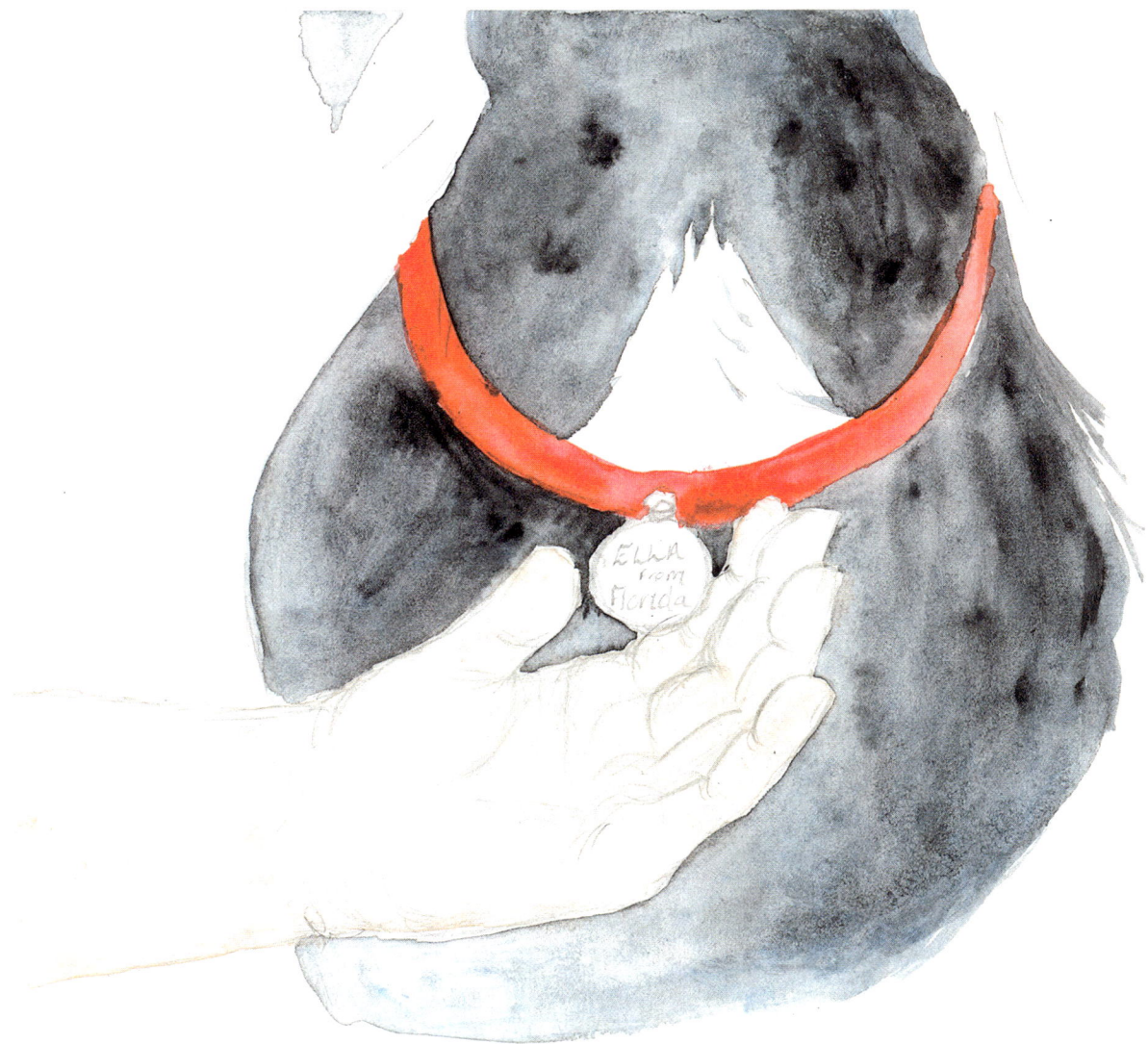

Hey, Ella, why don't you hop into my cart on top of this beautiful Alabama Crimson Tide stadium blanket. I keep it just for emergencies and this seems like an emergency," he said as he patted the blanket. Ella hopped up on it. She looked as if she had been through a long hard day and needed a rest.

Bill took out his phone and took a picture of Ella. His daughter, Emily, was a veterinarian and he wanted Emily to check Ella and make sure she was not hurt or sick. He sent Emily a message and a selfie with his new friend. Then Bill let Ella sleep while he waited for Emily to arrive.

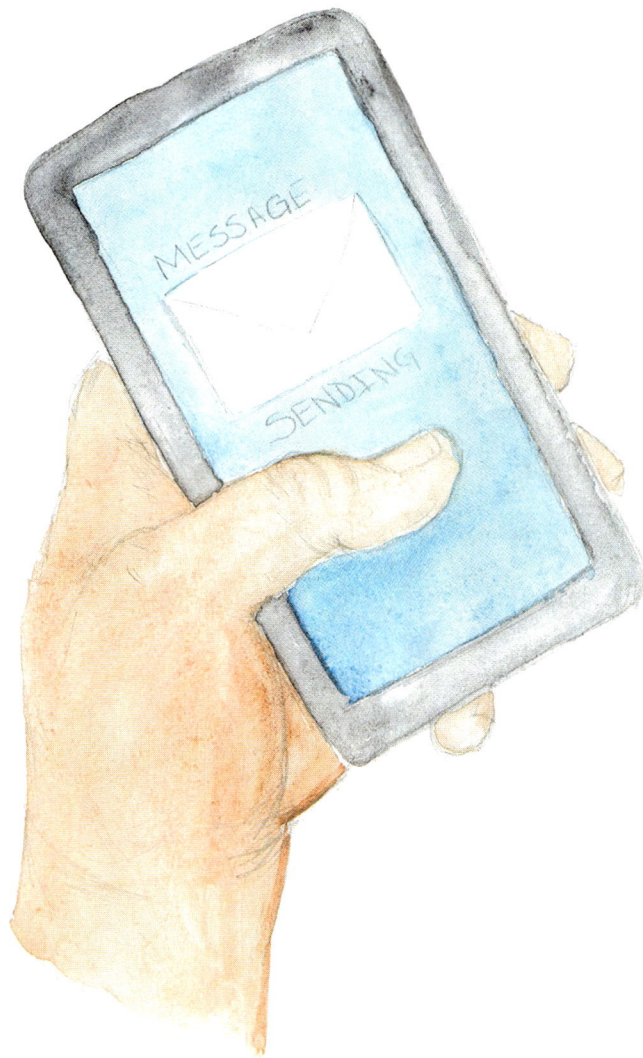

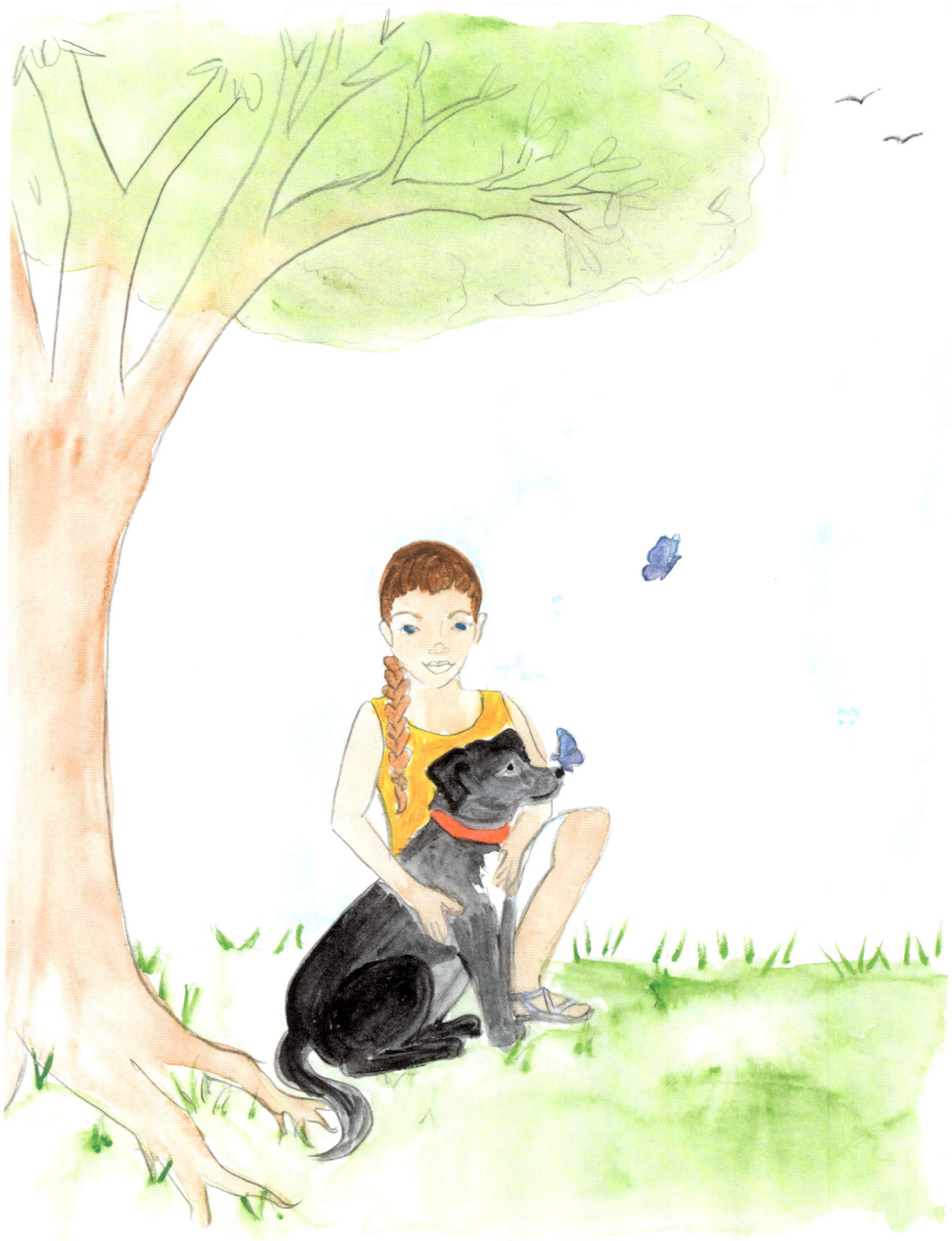

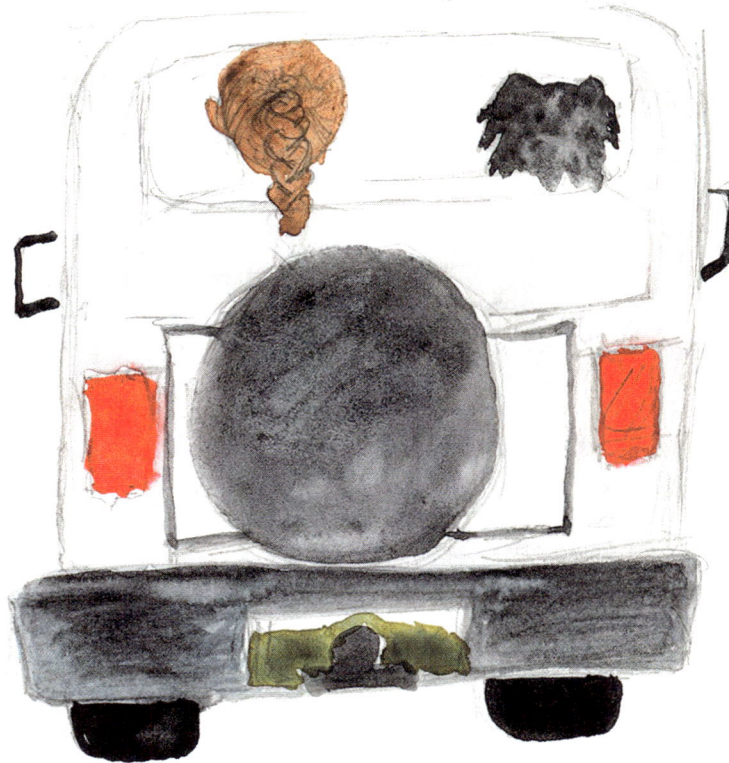

Emily knew her dad was a soft touch for animals and kids. But she knew he wouldn't ask for help if it wasn't needed. Emily was concerned for this new patient as she loaded food, water, bowls, toys, a blanket, and a leash into her Jeep. She climbed in and drove to meet her dad and Ella.

When Emily arrived at Dollywood, Ella climbed out of her dad's cart. Emily squatted down and lovingly greeted Ella, "What's up girl? You've had a long trip. How did you get here?"

Ella went to Emily and nudged her hand so that Emily would pet her. The two quickly became friends, and Ella jumped into the front seat as soon as Emily opened the door. Emily drove straight to the clinic.

When they arrived, Emily unlocked the door and let Ella in. In an exam room, Emily used the infrared scanner to find the chip in the back of Ella's neck. Emily gathered enough information so she could make a phone call later to a Sadie Middleton and try to solve the mystery of Ella's arrival at Dollywood.

Emily gently checked Ella's paws, ears, eyes, and heart rate. As she moved her hands over Ella's belly, Emily decided that an ultra sound was in order. Just as Emily had suspected, Ella was going to have puppies, five of them. Emily wondered how Ella had traveled so far. Ella did not seem to have been harmed by her trip.

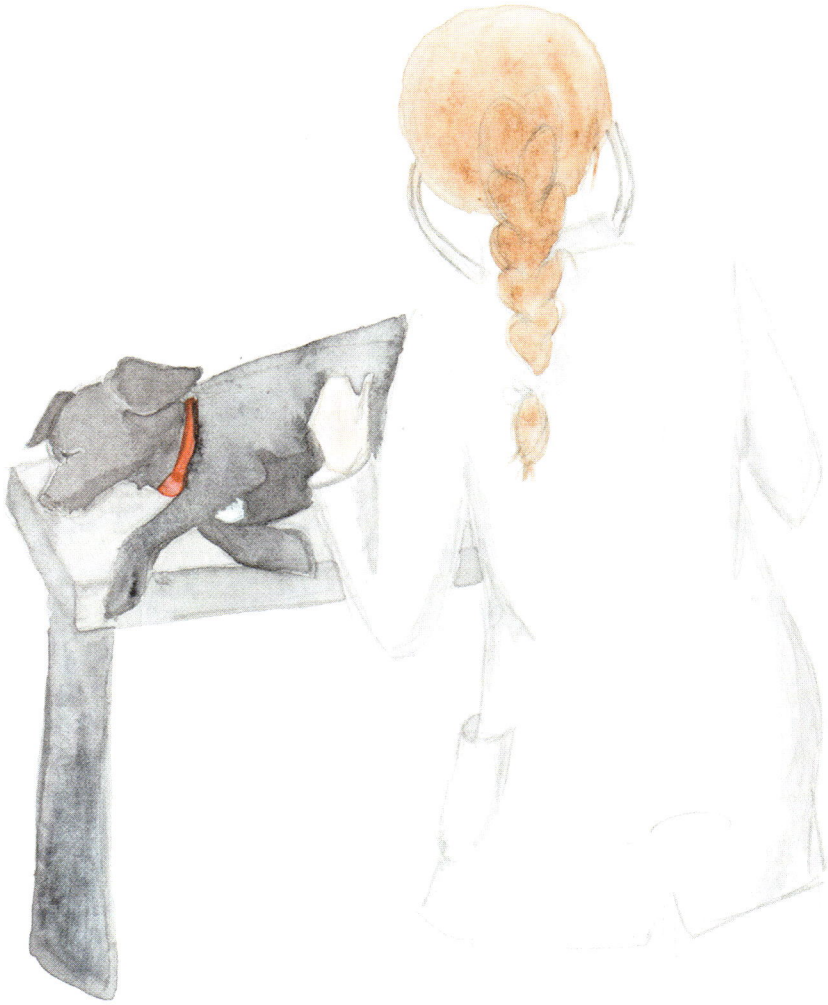

Emily took Ella home and introduced her to her 10-year-old daughter, Jordan. Jordan was thrilled to meet Ella. She ran to her and hugged her gently. Ella's tail was wagging and she seemed very happy to be with Jordan and Emily.

Jordan took Ella into the kitchen and offered her food and water saying, "You must be hungry and thirsty. I have exactly what you need." After Ella ate and drank, Jordan said, "Let's go out in the backyard to play? Jordan threw a ball to see if Ella would fetch. Not only would she fetch the ball, she was even able to catch it in her mouth.

Back in the kitchen where Emily was cooking their dinner, Jordan said, "I just knew that Ella was a great dog when I saw her, and she loves attention!"

After dinner and after Jordan and Ella had wrestled on the floor, and Jordan had read a book to Ella, Emily reminded her it was bedtime.

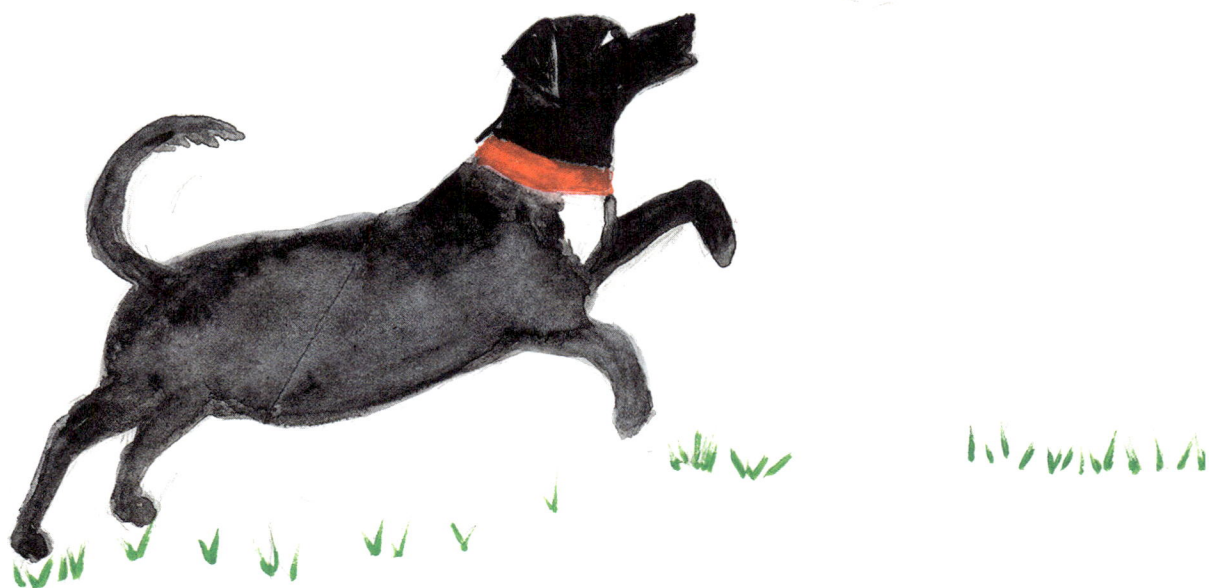

When Emily went in to tuck Jordan into bed, Ella was curled up on the end of Jordan's bed, already settled in for the night. Emily smiled and thought about how Sadie must be missing Ella. She wondered if Ella had curled up on Sadie's bed at night. Emily was glad that her dad had found Ella and that she was safe. Emily would call Florida in the morning.

Emily went into the kitchen and made herself a cup of tea. She called her dad and told him that Ella was going to have puppies and that she was a very lucky girl to be happy and healthy after such a long journey.

Emily went to bed but it was hard for her to sleep thinking about how Ella had traveled so far. She tossed and turned. It was a long night, without much rest. Normally she didn't take her patients' situations so hard, but something about Ella got to her. Ella seemed to be a well-loved, well-behaved, and loving dog. Emily wanted to know Ella's story, but she also was falling in love with Ella.

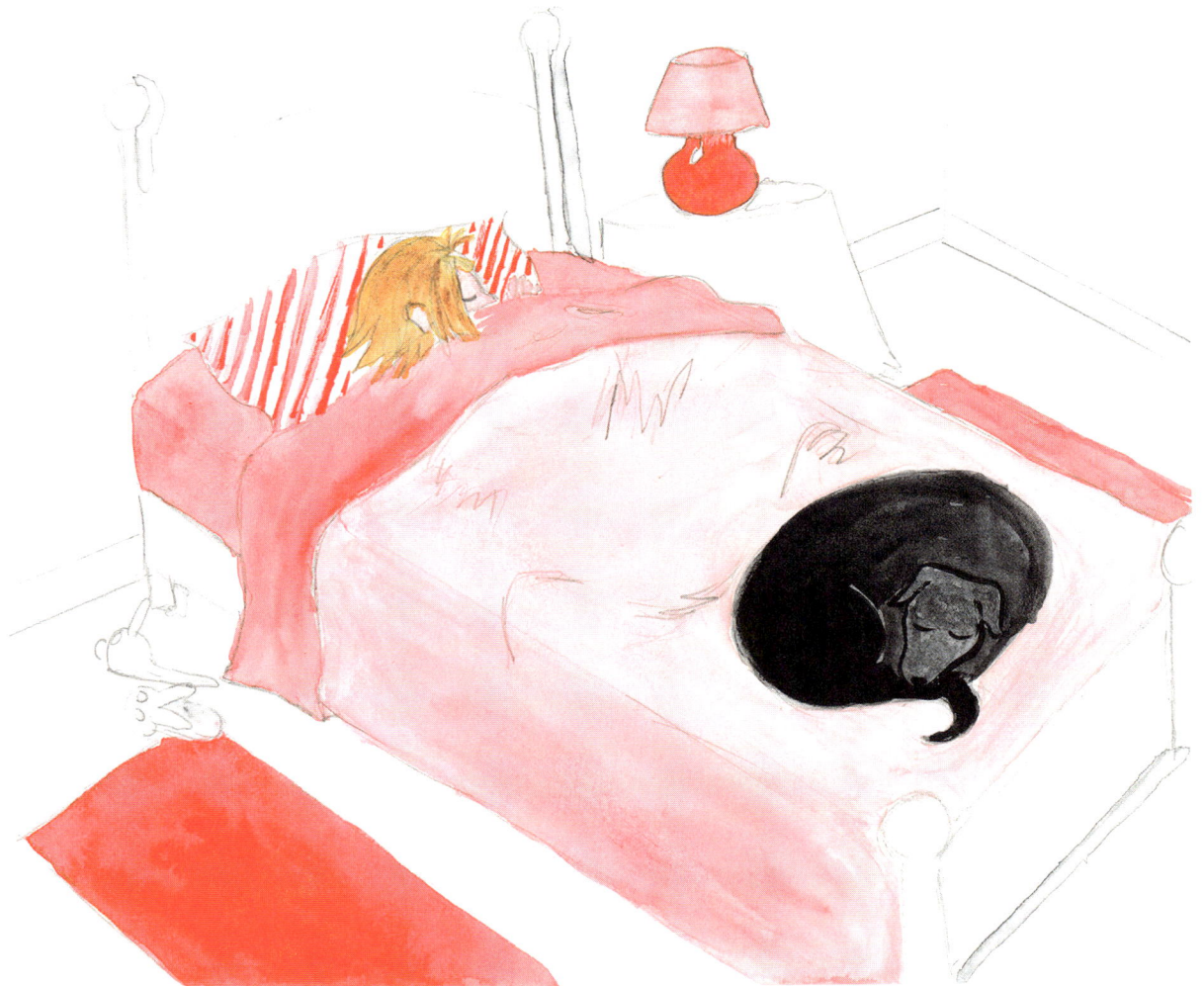

The next morning, Saturday, Emily woke up, made a pot of coffee, and then slipped into her jacket. She grabbed a leash and invited Ella to join her for a walk. Emily was really impressed with how well Ella obeyed commands.

When they walked back into the kitchen, Jordan had Ella's breakfast ready and fresh water waiting for her. Jordan asked, "Can I take Ella out back and play?"

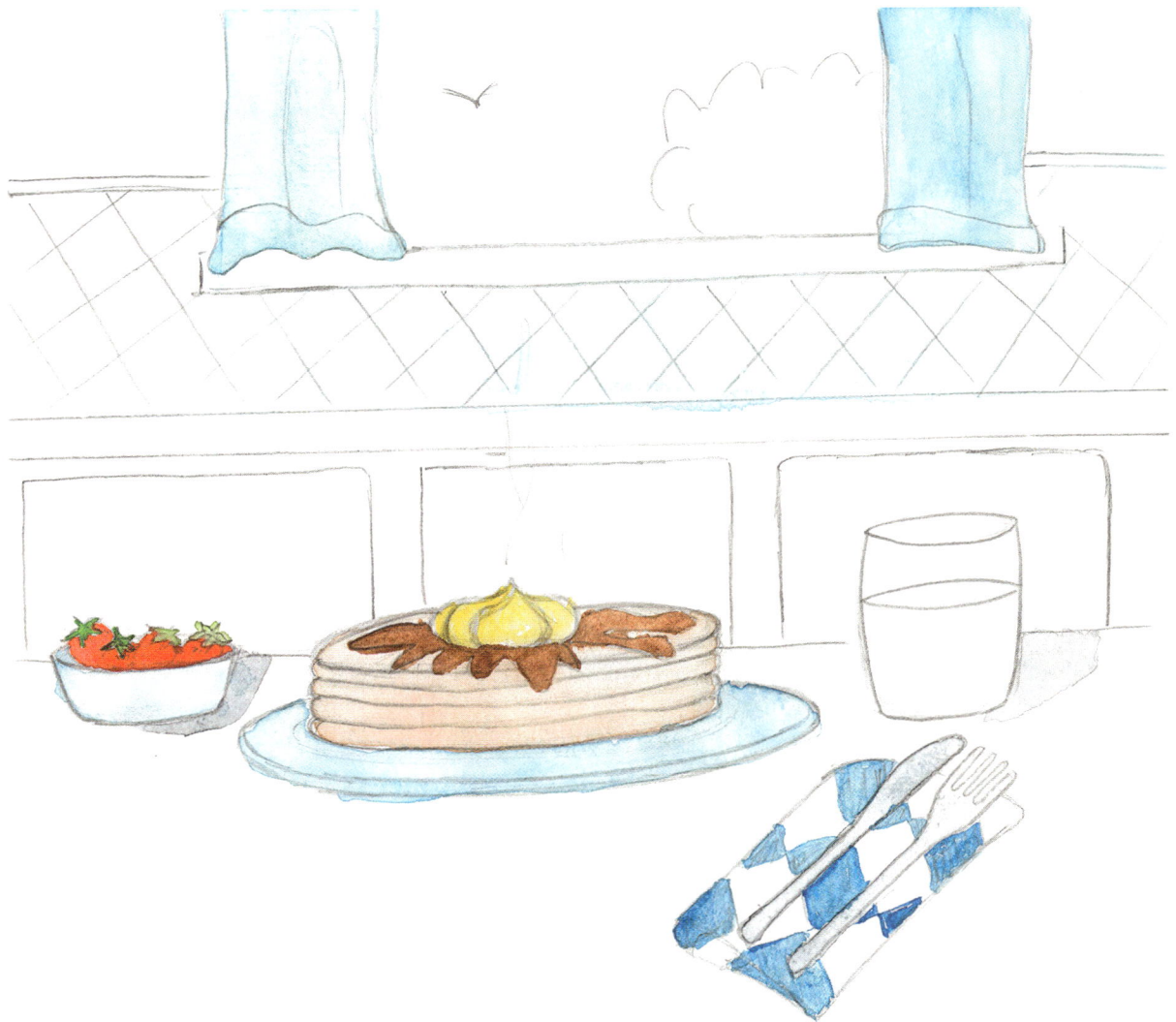

Emily answered, " That's fine, but only after you eat your breakfast and do your chores." Emily made Jordan pancakes with fruit and whipped cream.

After Jordan ate and put her dishes in the dishwasher, she made her bed, got dressed, and brushed her teeth. She pulled her hair up into a ponytail, took her dirty clothes to the laundry room, and grabbed her jacket. She was ready to start her day with her brand-new friend, Ella.

Emily smiled as Jordan and Ella headed out the back door. She grabbed the phone and punched in the number for Sadie in Florida. She quickly learned that Ella's owner, Sadie Middleton, had gone into a nursing home in Florence, Florida and could not keep Ella.

Sadie was surprised when Emily told her that she had Ella, but she was even more surprised when Emily said, "Ella is going to have five puppies."

Sadie explained, "My good friends, the Smallwoods, helped me move into my new home and they had taken Ella back to Michigan with them. I'm going to have to call the Smallwoods immediately, because they must surely be worried about Ella."

Sadie called the Smallwoods. Mrs. Smallwood cried and told Sadie, "Oh, we are so relieved, but we feel terrible that we had not told you Ella had been lost. We didn't want to upset you, so we have been searching for Ella on our own. We realized that she was missing around Pigeon Forge, Tennessee, so we have been posting about Ella on Facebook. We called every veterinary office in the area, but we haven't heard anything yet."

Sadie told Mrs. Smallwood, "Ella is pregnant. She is having five puppies."

Mrs. Smallwood then began to cry. "Oh, I am so sorry, Sadie, but there is simply no way we can care for Ella and five puppies, too."

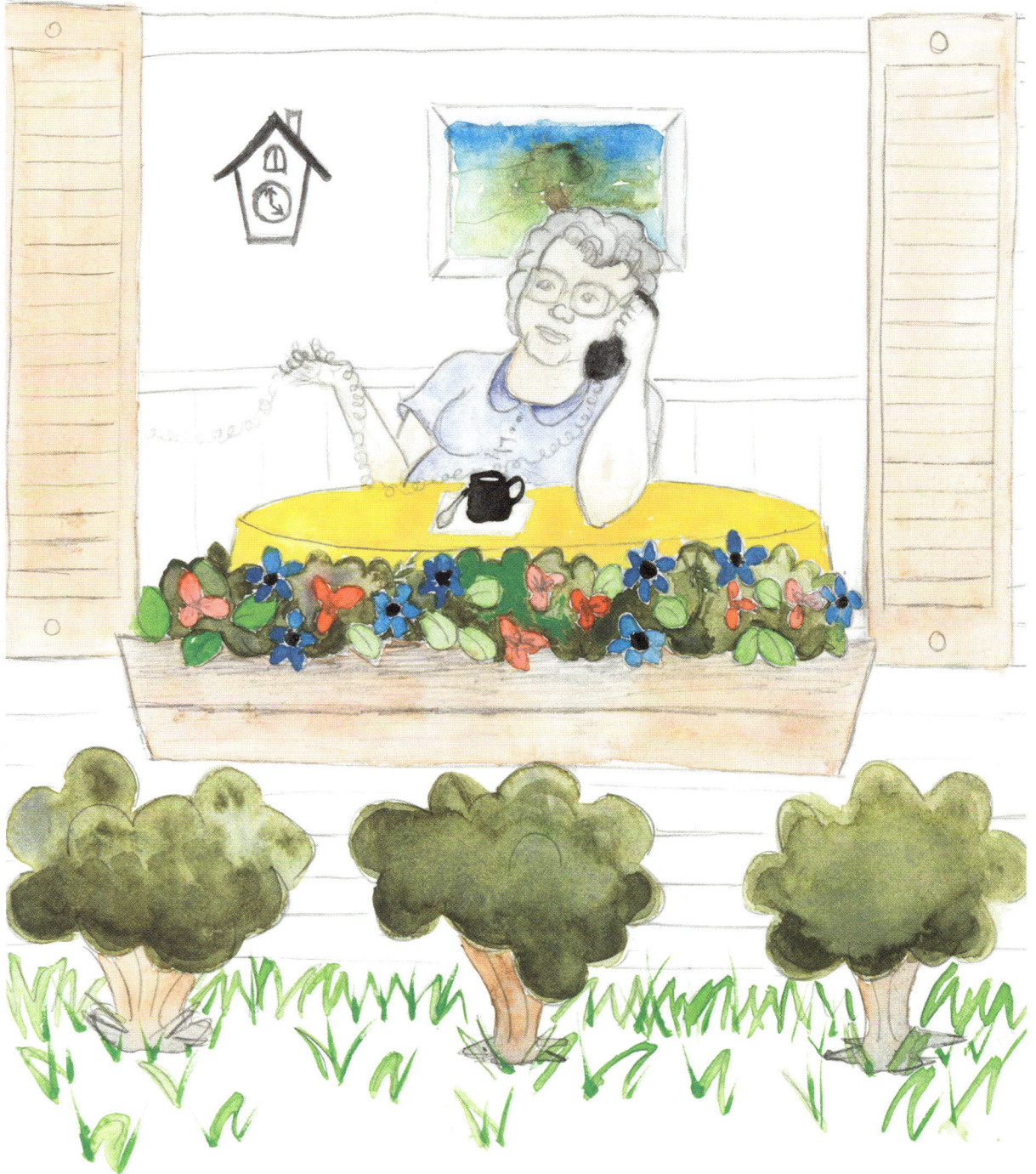

Sadie called Emily and told her about her conversation with Mrs. Small-wood. Sadie quietly said she was not sure what to do. Emily told Sadie, " I have the perfect solution. My daughter, Jordan, has been begging me for a dog. When I went to tuck Jordan in bed last night, Ella was curled up at the end of Jordan's bed. Right now, they are outside playing as we talk. Jordan has already fallen in love with Ella. Truth be told, so have I."

Sadie was so happy to know that Ella was loved that she cried. They agreed to keep in touch and said good-bye.

Emily then called her dad, and told him, "Jordan has a new pet, thanks to you." She shared how the Smallwoods had lost track of Ella in Pigeon Forge. "Oh, Dad, I am so thankful that Ella had stayed safe and you found her. Now Jordan is so happy to have Ella. You know she has been begging me to let her have a pet.

"I also have an idea about how to help other people with Ella's puppies."

Emily and Jordan went shopping for a new collar and leash for Ella at the pet store, then they took Ella to the dog park. She played fetch with a ball and caught a Frisbee in her mouth. Jordan was so happy to have Ella as a friend. Emily knew that she and Jordan loved Ella already.

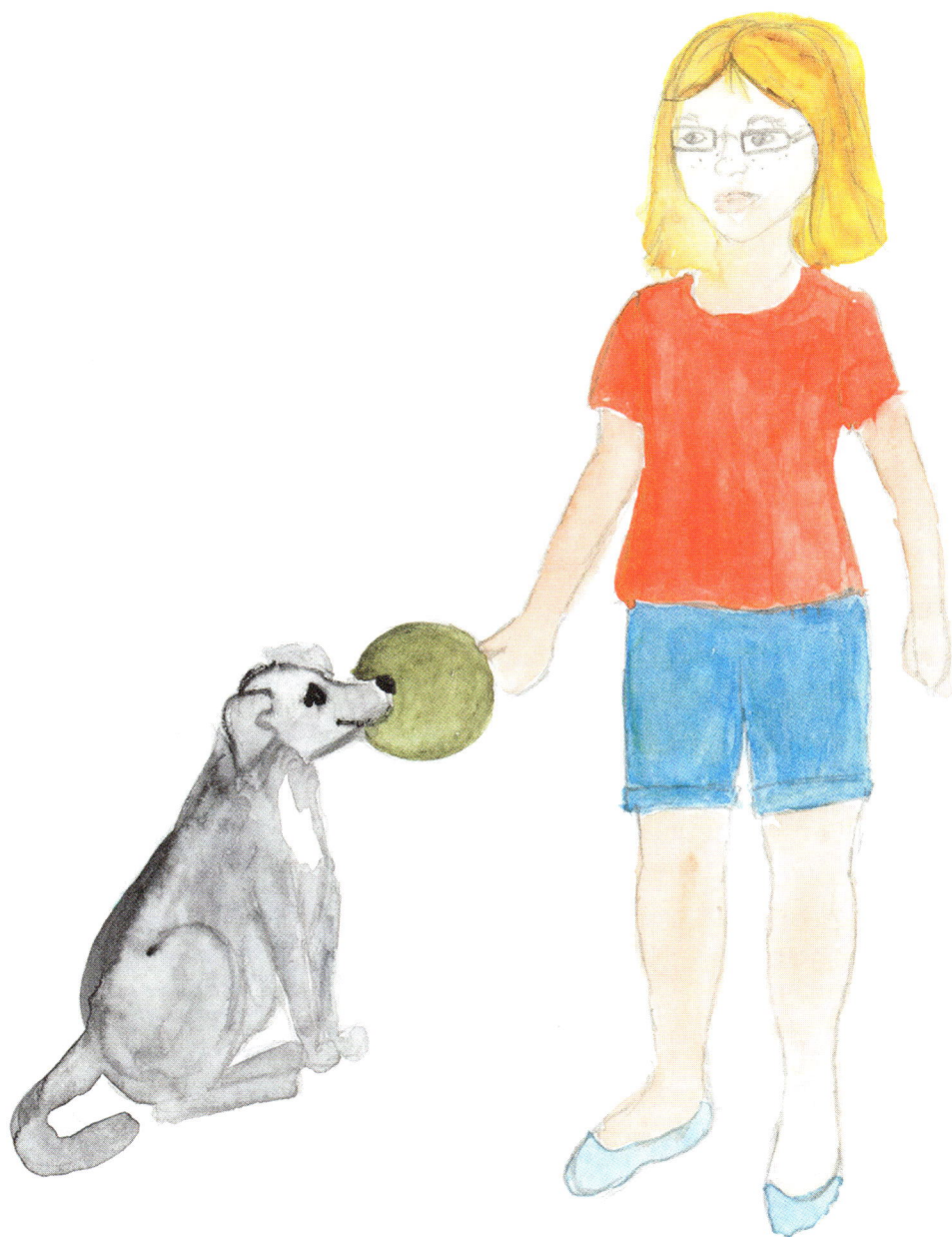

Monday morning Emily called Wilderwood Service Dogs in Maryville, Tennessee to ask if it would be possible to try to work with Ella's puppies to become service dogs. Tiffany said that they could give it a try. Tiffany explained that dogs can start to be trained as soon as they are ready to leave their mother, around 8-9 weeks, and training takes about a year.

Tiffany said she uses a puppy development tool call puppy neuro-stimulation. This helps the puppies grow to their full potential and Emily needed to learn how to do this. It was actually very easy. She needed to pick up each puppy, twice a day and gently (cradling them in her hand) turn them sideways, backwards and then forwards. She also needed to touch them all over, in between their toes and behind their ears, everywhere while talking softly to them.

Tiffany suggested that Emily look into foster homes for dogs in training. They would need people to work with them on basic commands like sit, down, wait, potty, come. They would learn their name as well and how to behave appropriately on a leash. Until the dogs went for actual service dog training, Jordan and Emily would need to play with them, brush them and take them for walks. The most important thing that the puppies would need was to socialize with people and other dogs.

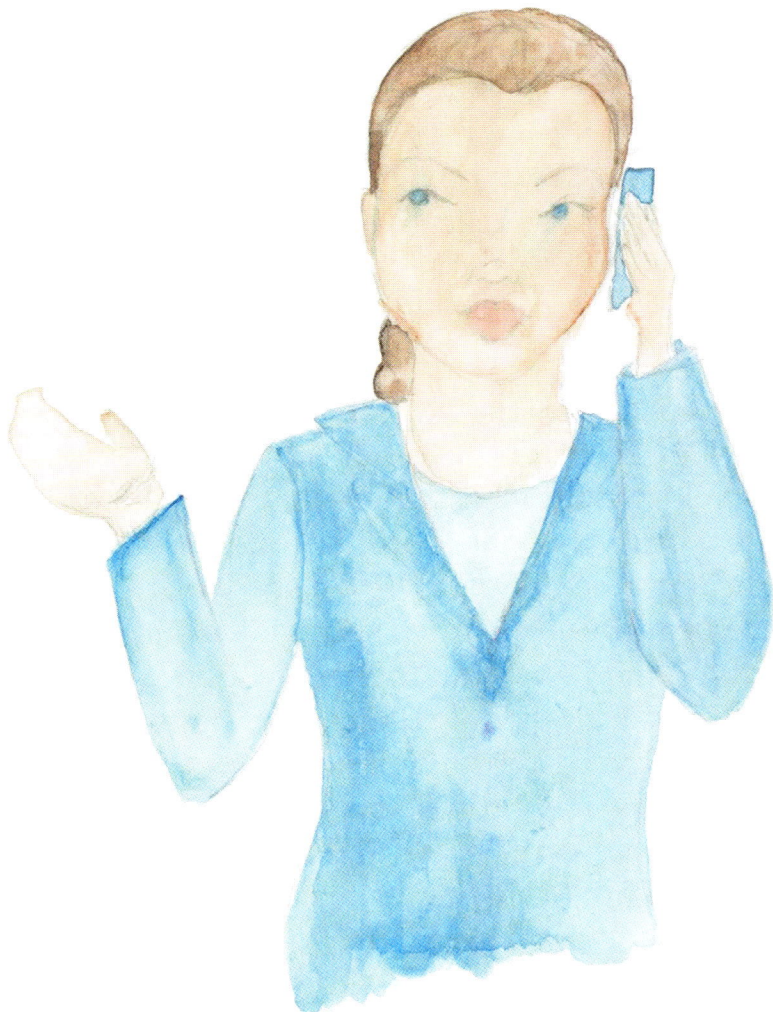

Jordan and Emily cared for Ella and got everything ready for the puppies to be born. On a bright sunny day in May, Ella began whimpering and acting different than usual. Emily knew that she was going to have her puppies soon. Emily brought home a whelping box from the clinic for Ella to have the puppies in. She put the box in a dark corner of her bedroom and turned on some very soft music. She took Ella outside to potty a few times and then Ella let Emily know that it was time for the puppies to be born.

As Ella gave birth to her puppies, instinct took over; she knew just what to do. She cleaned and looked over each one from head to toe. She lovingly gathered her babies up close until all five were lined up and nursing. It was only when all the work was done that Ella rested as she fed her puppies. Jordan slept through the delivery. When she woke up in the morning, there were five beautiful little pups snuggled up to Ella. Emily had checked the puppies and knew that they were all healthy. Ella had two boys and three girls. Jordan looked on and thought of names for Ella's family. Krystal was light brown, Rocky was black and brown, Snowflake was white with a few brown spots, Annie was golden brown, and Manny was black. They were beautiful. Ella was proud of her puppies. She took very good care of them.

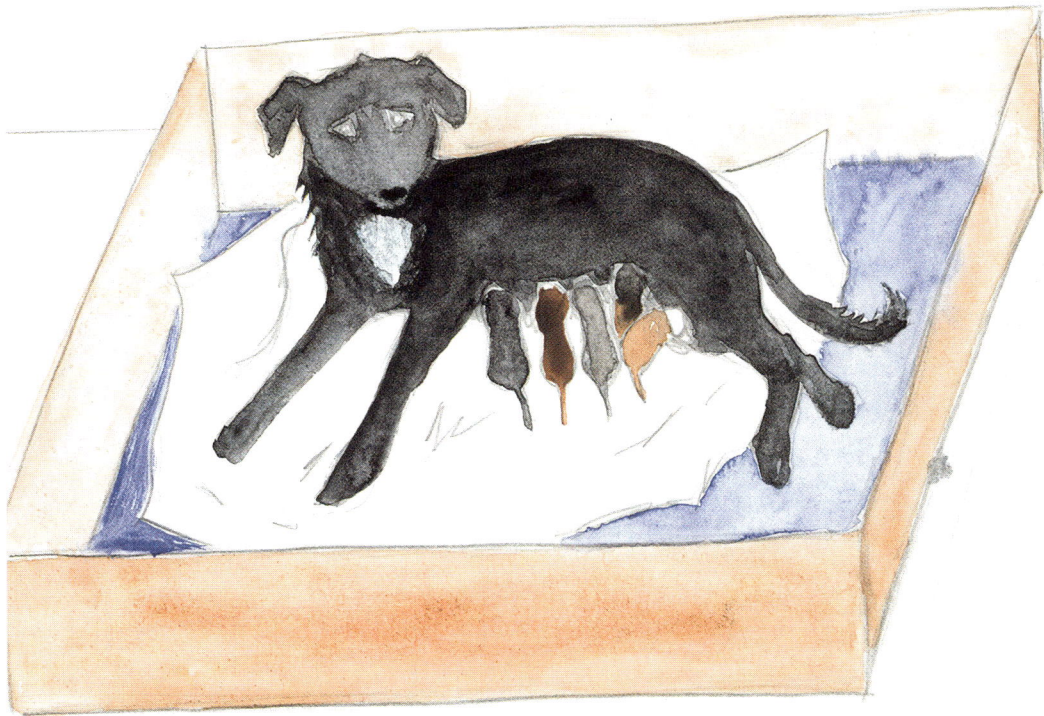

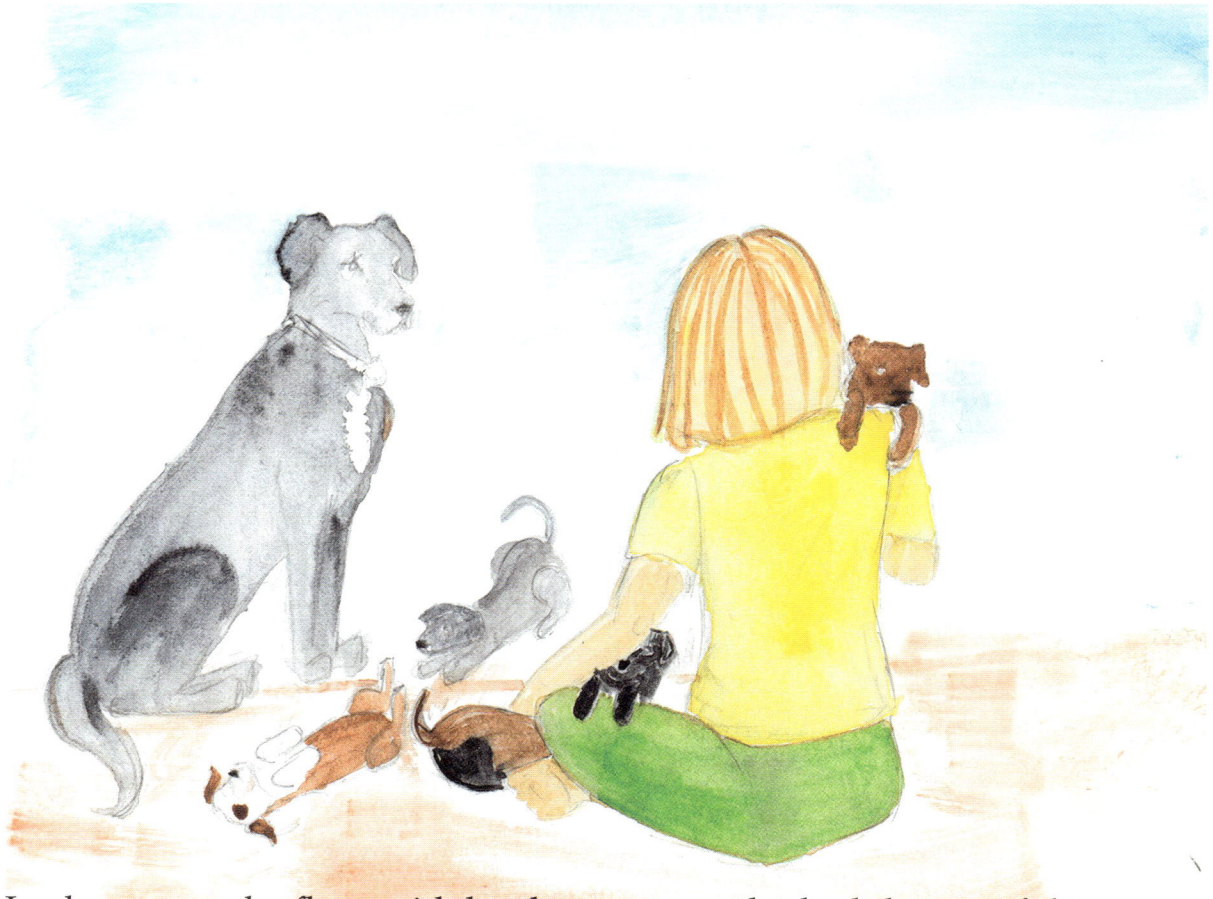

Jordan sat on the floor with her legs outstretched while two of the puppies jumped onto her lap and tumbled over each other. Two chased each other's tails, while one nibbled on her toes. Jordan petted them, crawled around letting them follow her, then lay flat out on the floor while they gave her puppy kisses and tugged at her clothes. They would back up, give a little bark and lunge at her. She had never even imagined anything being this fun. She loved Ella and her puppies so much. When Ella thought they had played long enough, she rounded them up and put them to bed.

By the middle of June, the puppies had begun eating solid food and were ready to leave Ella. Nichole, the trainer at Wilderwood, had worked with Jordan on basic commands and they were getting those down. As they started to leave for their foster homes, it was so hard for Jordan to say goodbye. She wondered if Ella really understood that people would be taking her babies, one by one. It made her cry sometimes.

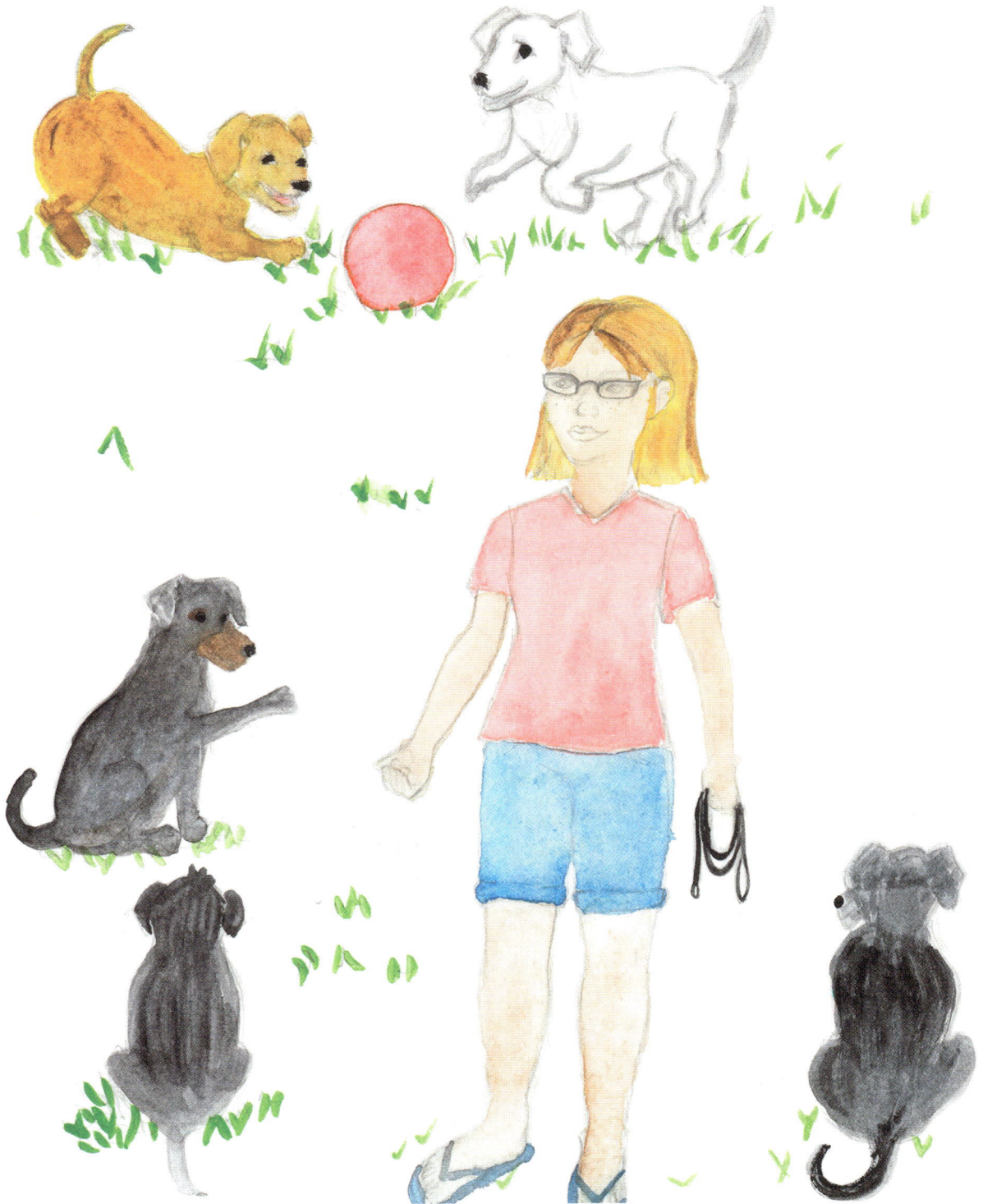

She was thankful that Ella was her dog, and she could still see the puppies now and then, but she knew that she would miss them so much.

Tom and Julie Baker came Saturday morning with their daughter Rachel. Rachel was 12 and she understood that Krystal was going to be with them for training. She had already read all of the paperwork and promised to walk Krystal, feed her, and work with her every day. She would be taking Krystal out to different places to get comfortable because that would be Krystal's job when she graduated from training. Jordan talked to Rachel and hoped that they might become friends. They both lived in Pigeon Forge, and went to the same school. They agreed to meet at the park with the dogs every few weeks. Jordan felt ok about the first puppy going home with the Bakers. She hoped that Ella felt the same.

Jordan took the other puppies outside and played with them. She worked with them, one at a time, on the simple commands. They were doing very well. Jordan and Emily were very proud of the puppies.

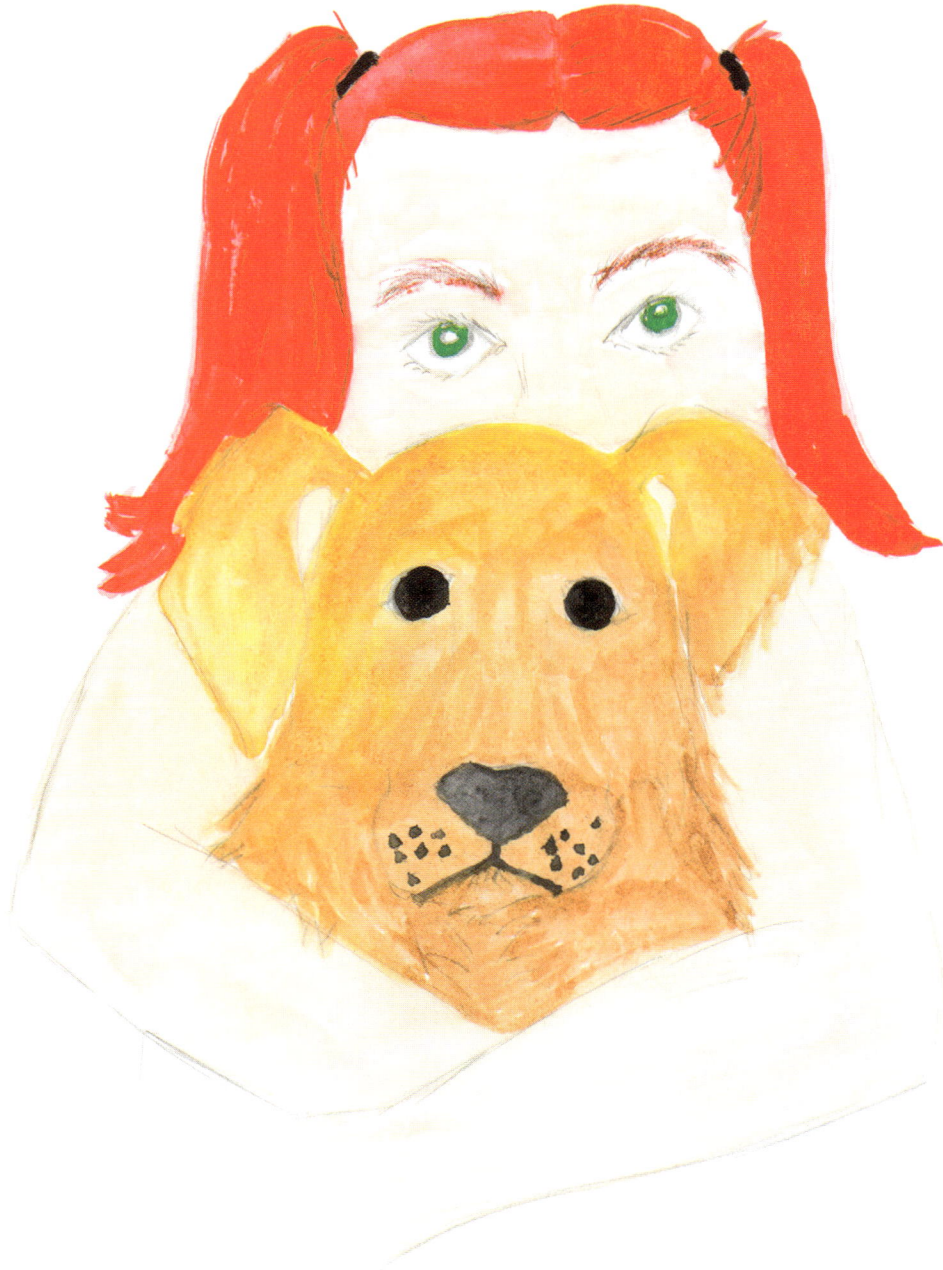

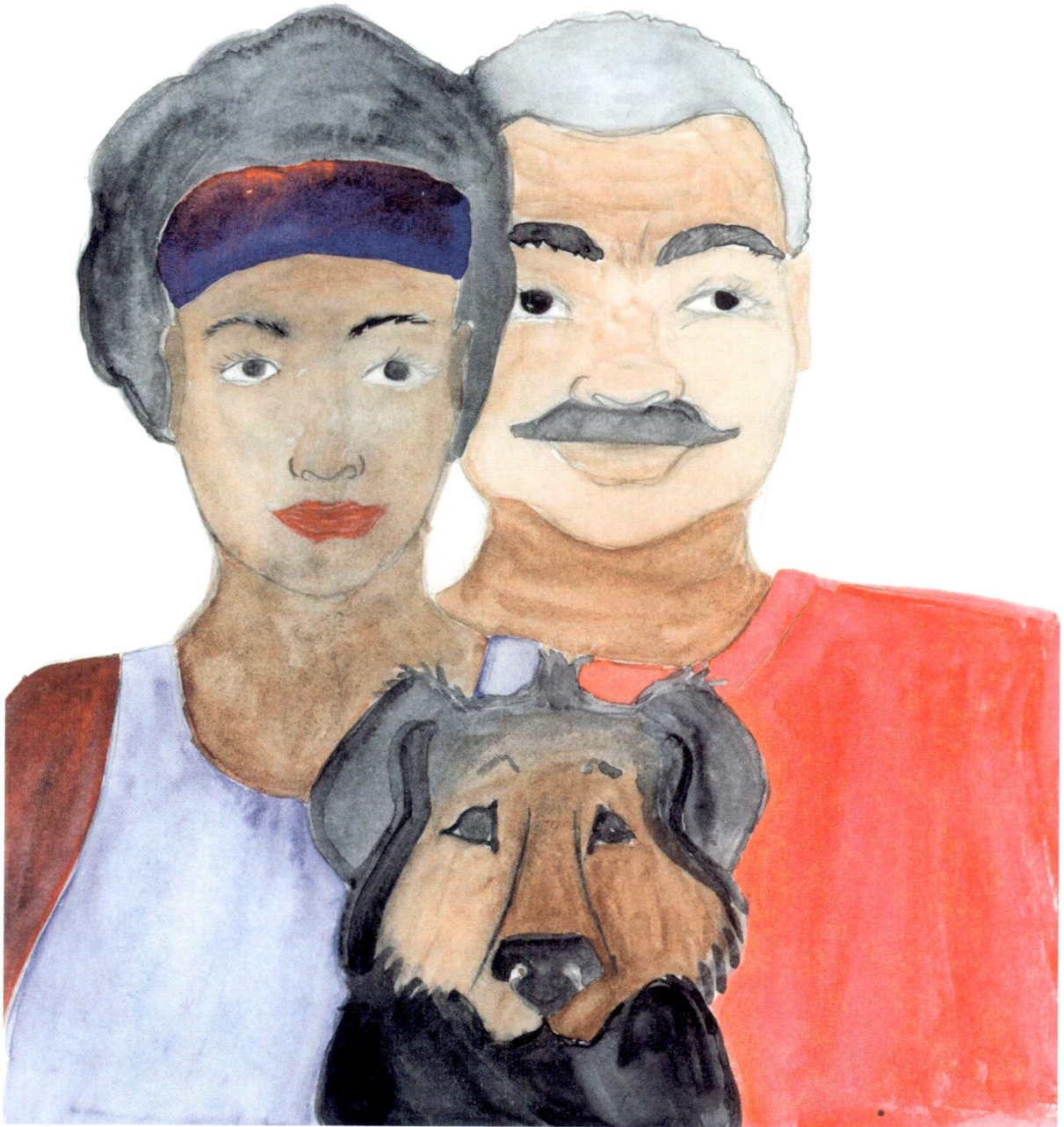

Tuesday morning, Jordan met the Thompsons when they came to pick up Rocky. Janet and Burt didn't have children living at home. Their children were grown and lived in other parts of the country. They were both retired and felt excited about having a puppy to be responsible for. They lived in Gatlinburg, which was not far from Pigeon Forge. Again, Jordan did not like saying goodbye, but it was something she knew that she had to do. Taking care of all of the puppies was getting to be a big job.

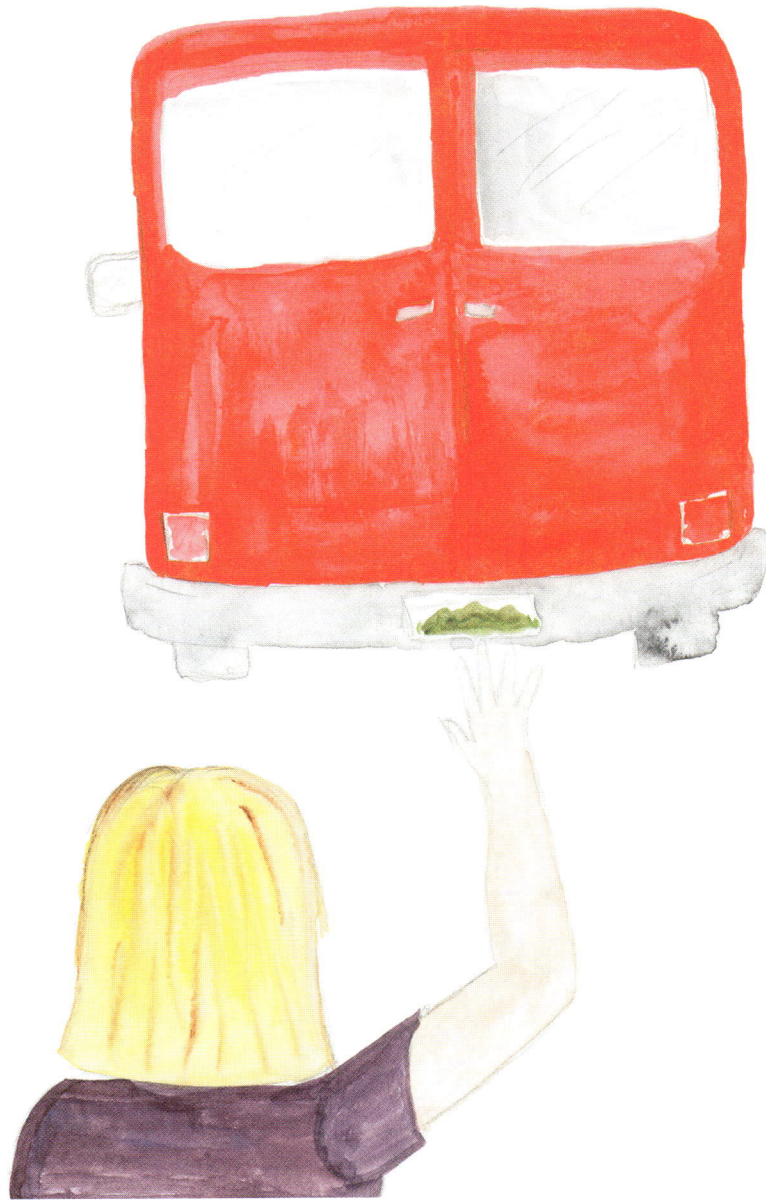

Wednesday evening before dinner, the Browns came with their five children. They played in the yard with Jordan, Ella, and her three remaining puppies while Ike and Mindy spoke to Emily. Selina, Stacy, Roy, Stanley, and Regina were homeschooled. Taking care of Snowflake was a way that their parents thought would help them learn responsibility. Ike and Mindy thought this was a great way to help them learn something very important while helping at the same time.

The kids were nice, but there sure were a lot of them! Jordan was used to being the only kid at her house. She wondered how they would divide the chores and training for Snowflake. She hoped that one of them would love Snowflake as much as she did. She waved goodbye as they loaded into their big van and headed back to their home in Kodak.

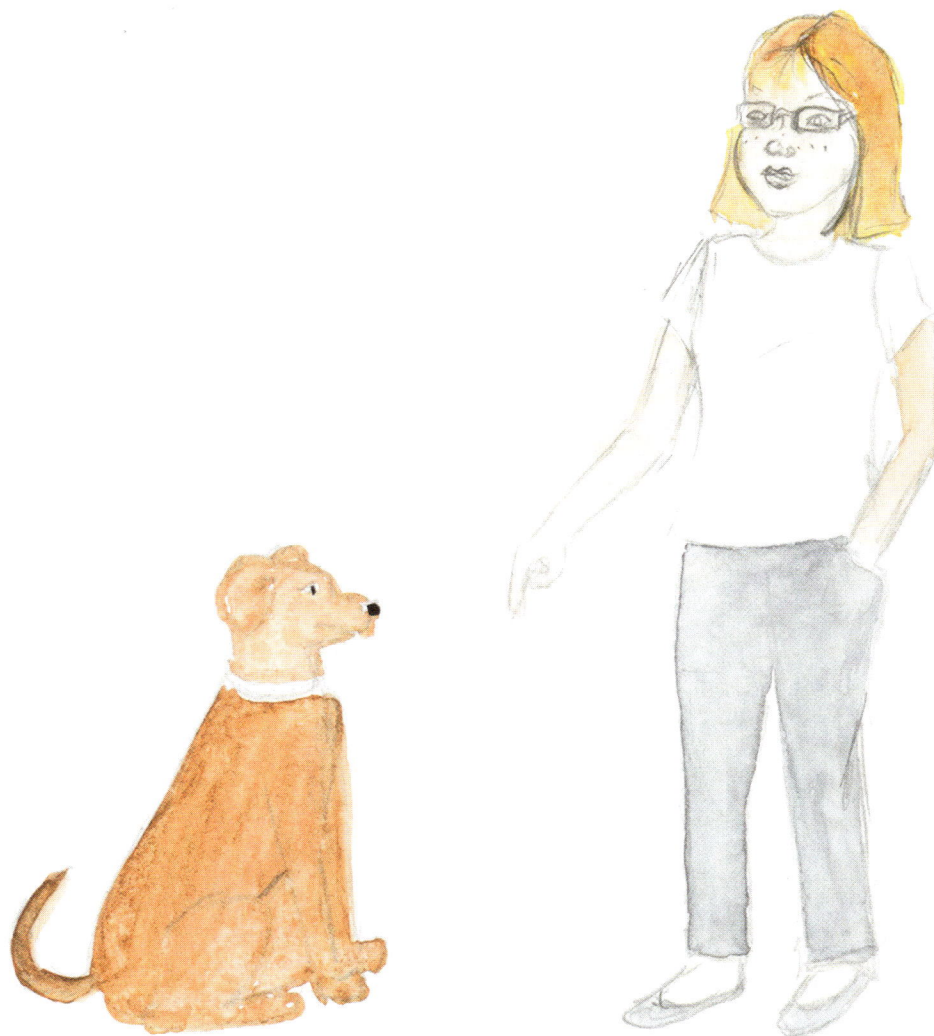

Friday afternoon Gabe and Bonnie Jackson arrived with their three children, Timothy, Sarah, and Chloe. They were there for Annie. They lived in Alcoa, very near the service dog agency. Timothy and Sarah were teenagers and Jordan thought they would take great care of Annie. She hoped they would, because secretly Annie was her favorite puppy. She loved them all, but next to Ella she was most partial to Annie. Jordan demonstrated all the commands that Annie knew and then gathered up her leash and dishes.

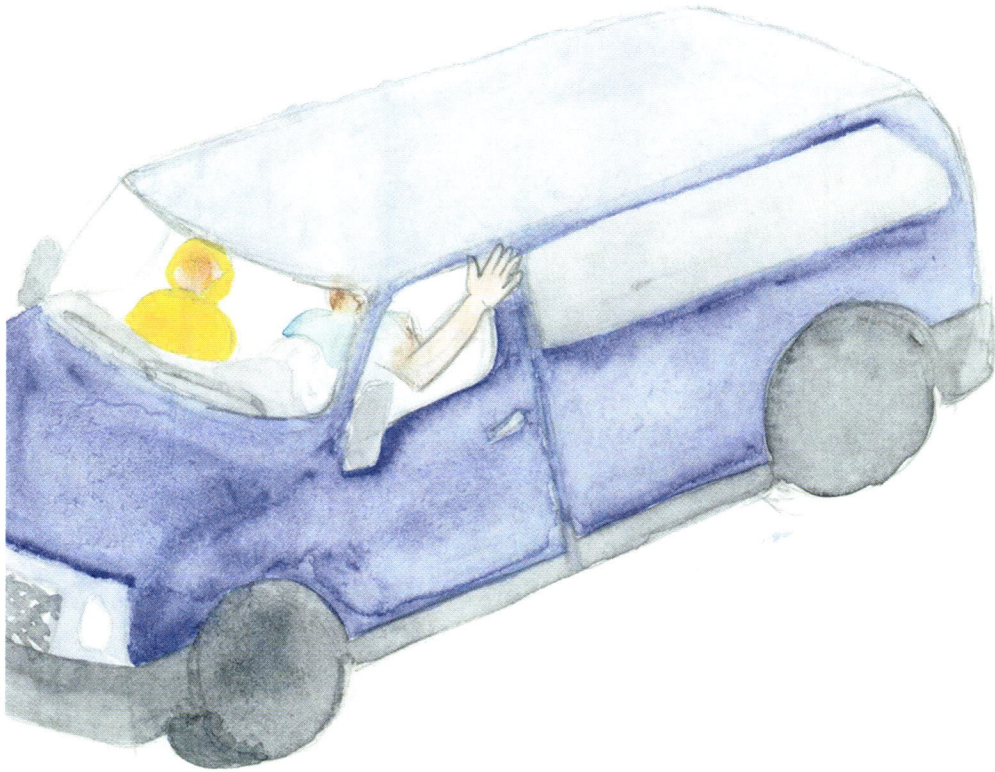

Emily took dogfood out to their van. Little Chloe smiled and waved as her dad buckled her into her car seat. She kept saying, "Sit Annie," as the puppy climbed onto Sarah's lap. Jordan waved through tears. It was getting harder.

Saturday came too soon. Jenny and Henry Fox arrived with their twins, Michael and Michelle. They were 11 and Jordan knew them from baseball. They would take Manny to their home in Maryville. Manny looked the most like Ella, although his actions were nothing like his mom. Jordan walked them through the commands and they watched quietly, then each repeated what Jordan had modeled for them. Jordan thought that all of Ella's puppies were in good hands. Why then, she wondered, was her heart so heavy? Why did she sit down and cry after they left?

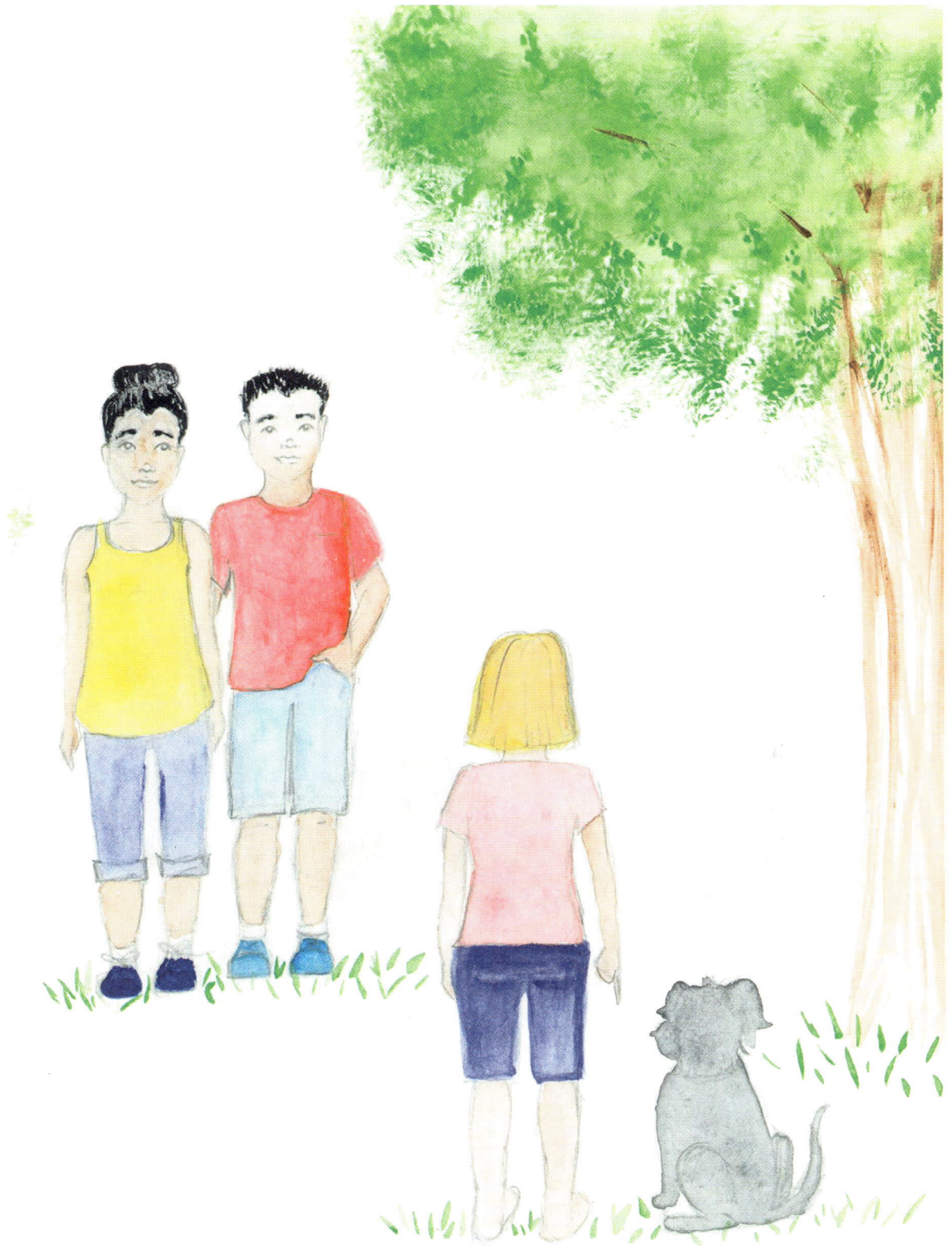

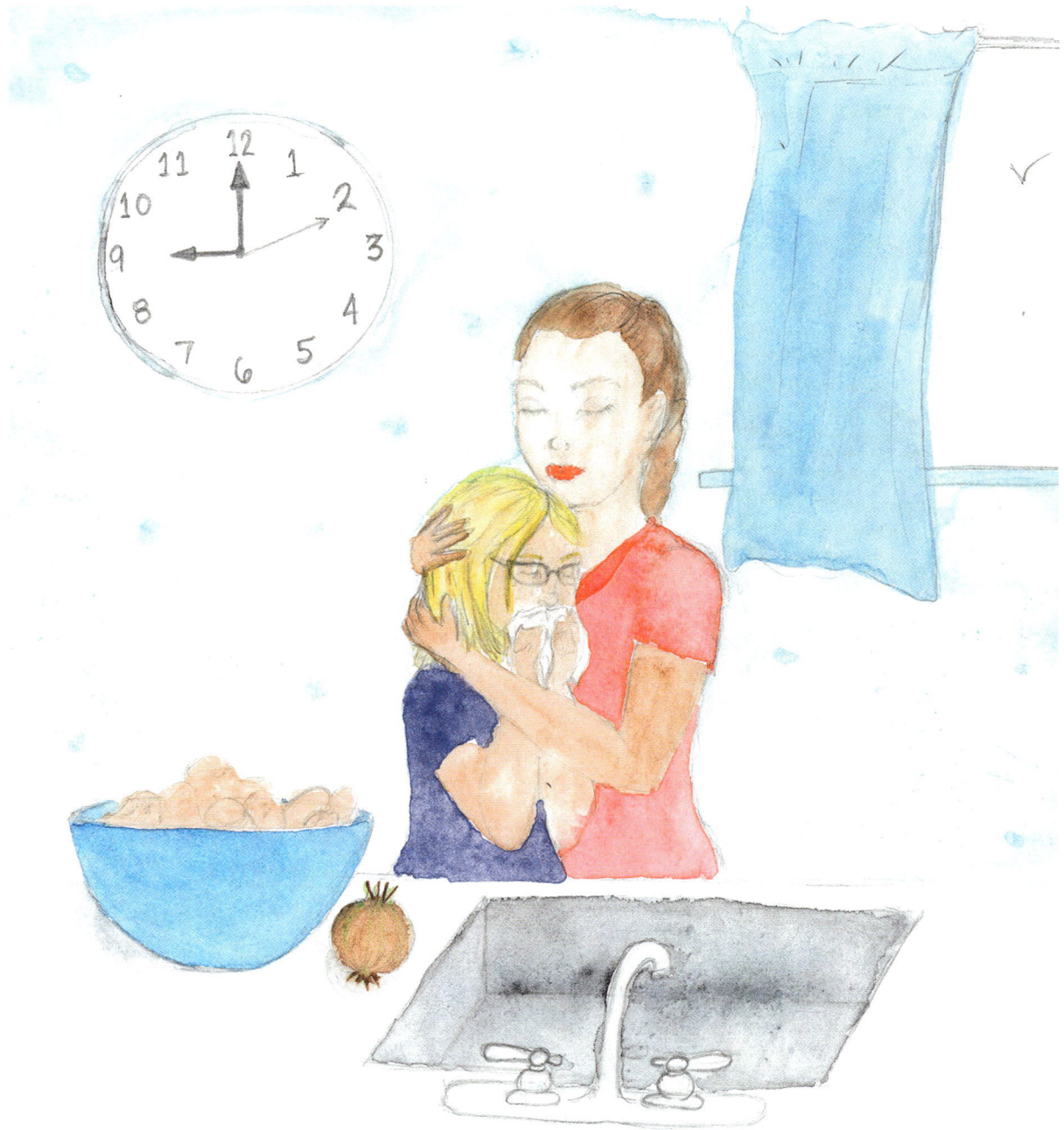

Emily hugged her daughter. "Remember how amazing it is that so many people will be blessed by Ella and her puppies."

"Mom, I know, but it doesn't help me feel better right now with all of the puppies gone to their new homes. I miss them. Ella must miss them, too."

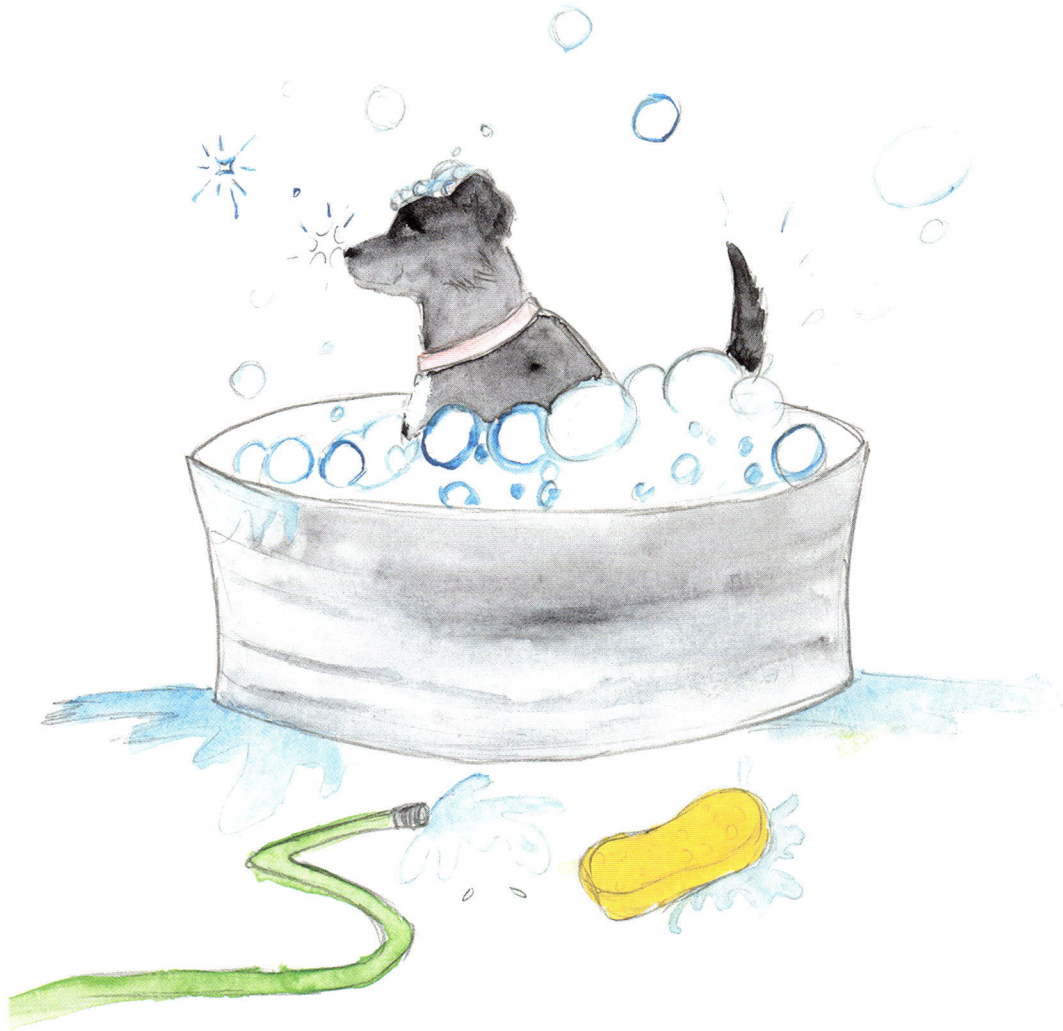

"Oh, Jordan, I miss them terribly too, but now we have to make potato salad for the family reunion Sunday afternoon."

Jordan helped her mother in the kitchen and then took Ella out for a long walk. It seemed like Ella was sad too. Jordan decided to give Ella lots of attention so she would not miss her puppies so much. She gave Ella a bath and brushed her Then she needed a bath herself!

Ella was dry by the time Jordan climbed into bed. Emily looked in on them and thought of that first night that Ella had come to them. So much had changed since that night. So much love had multiplied and so many lives had changed. So many lives were going to be touched in the future.

Emily and Jordan packed up the jeep after church and headed for Douglas Dam. Emily was excited to see her grandparents since they had just gotten back from a trip out west. Jordan was excited to see her cousins and tell them about Ella and her puppies. She hoped that her uncle Jack had brought his boat.

She was ready to go for a ride, and she hoped that Jack wouldn't mind another passenger. She wondered if they might have a life jacket for Ella. She smiled inside when she thought of Ella's ears flapping in the breeze as they pulled her cousins behind them on a tube. This was going to be a great day!

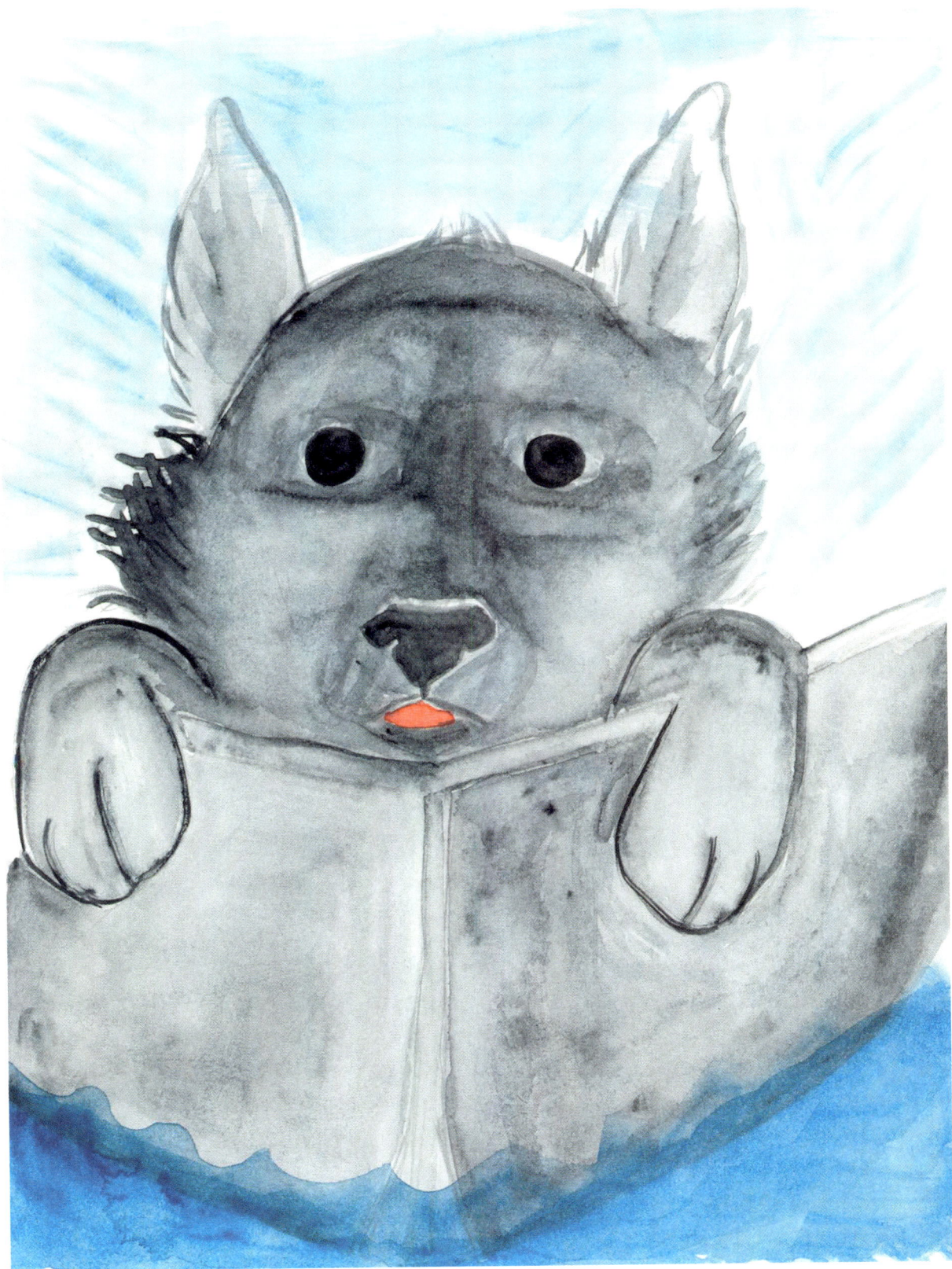

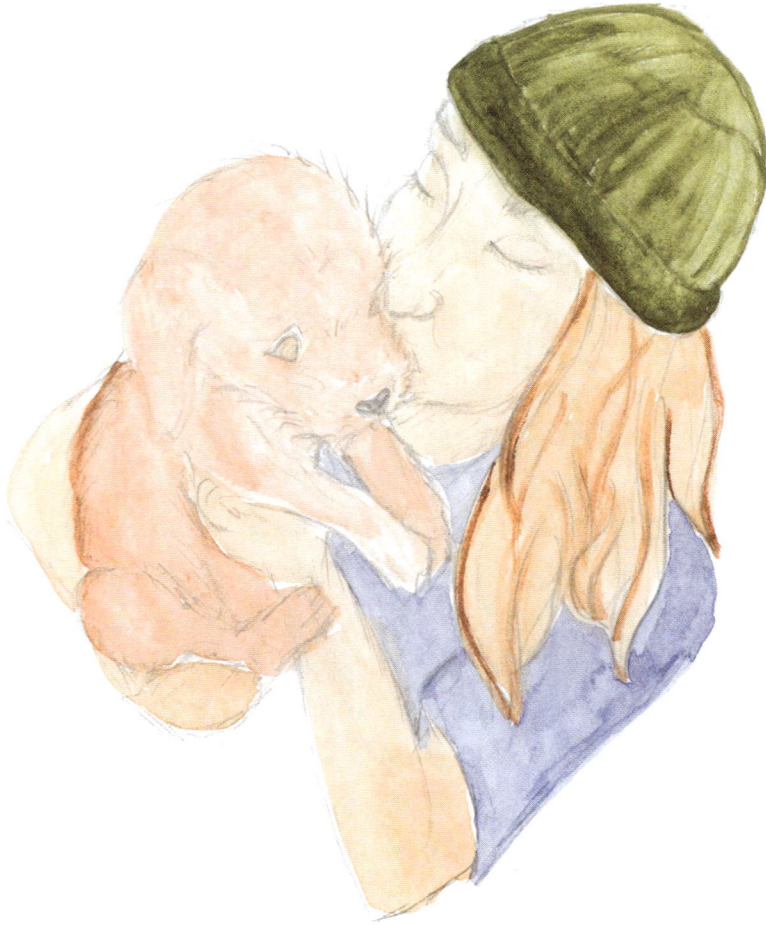

The foster families were amazing. They worked closely with Nichole to help the puppies with socializing and obeying commands. The puppies grew and became well-mannered dogs. They played ball and chewed on their toys, but they knew when they were expected to do their jobs. A harness is used when they are on duty, which is a cue for the dog but also allows people to understand that it is not time for them to play.

They started going out with their prospective owners in the fall. Nichole taught them ways to best help their person.

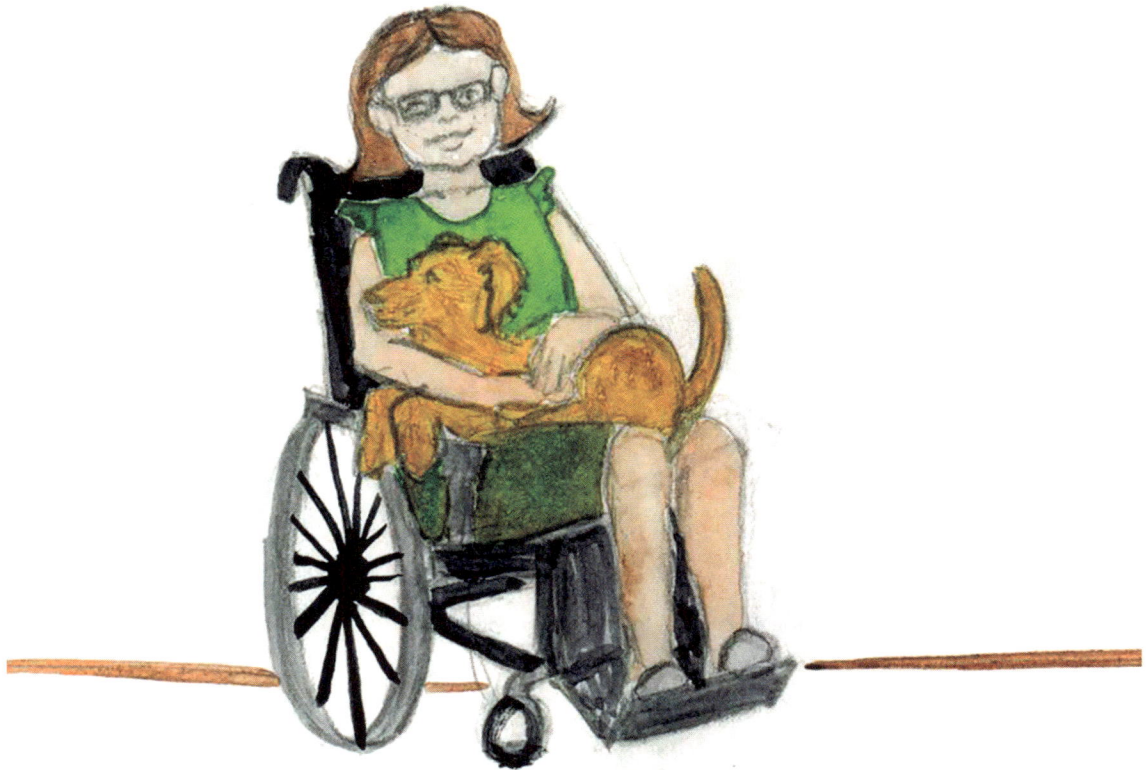

Angel spends her days in a wheelchair because she has Spina Bifida. She doesn't feel much from the waist down, and cannot walk at all since her back surgery. Angel has to depend on her parents and her sisters to help her with almost everything. She loves art and crafts, and is great with her hands, but when it came to playing outside on the playground, Angel felt left out and anxious. When Krystal came into Angel's life she had so much more freedom. Krystal could open doors and retrieve items as Angel requested. Krystal could assist her with chores and undressing, putting things away and helping her get around. It was great to have a friend that she could count on that never left her side. Krystal even slept by Angel at night in case she needed something. There were dozens of commands that Krystal could still learn to help Angel. They continued training together and they quickly became best friends.

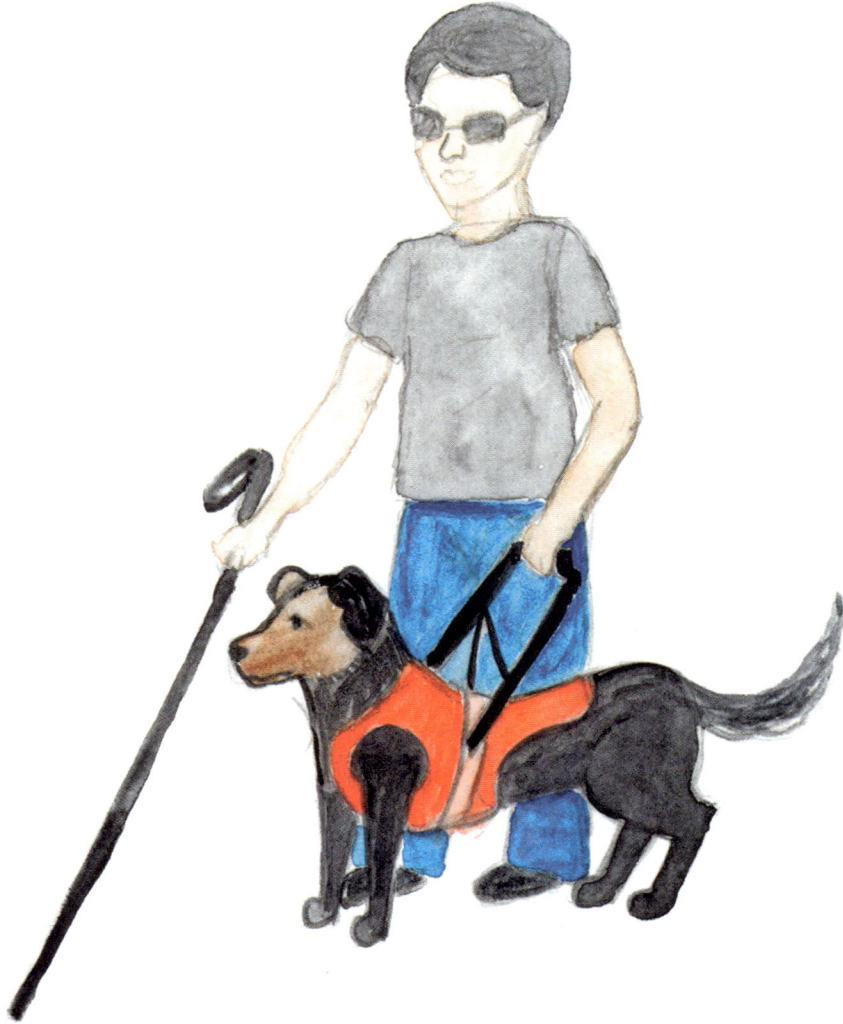

Timothy was blind, so Rocky had to be his eyes and keep him safe. Timothy had lost his sight after an accident at 19, so Rocky had to help Timothy stay calm as well. It was hard for Timothy to get around when he could no longer see. Nichole assured him that Rocky would be his best friend and help him maneuver through life.

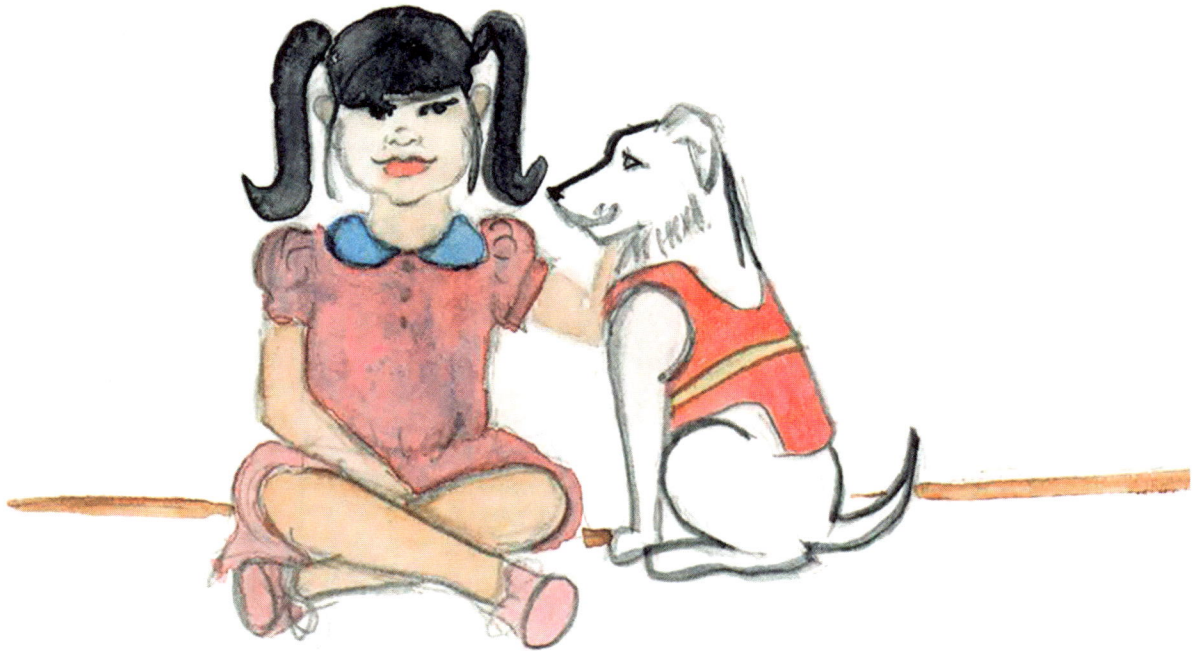

Lilly looked like any other five-year-old little girl. She was different in that she was adopted from China so she looked different from her parents. Just meeting her, you could not see her disability. Snowflake, or Snow as the Brown family had lovingly started calling her, would keep Lilly safe if she was about to have a seizure. Lilly had Epilepsy. Sometimes she would fall during a seizure and her parents worried that she might get hurt. Snow would let Lilly know before a seizure began so she could get to a safe place and she would stay with her and then snuggle with her when she woke up. Lilly always felt safe with Snow.

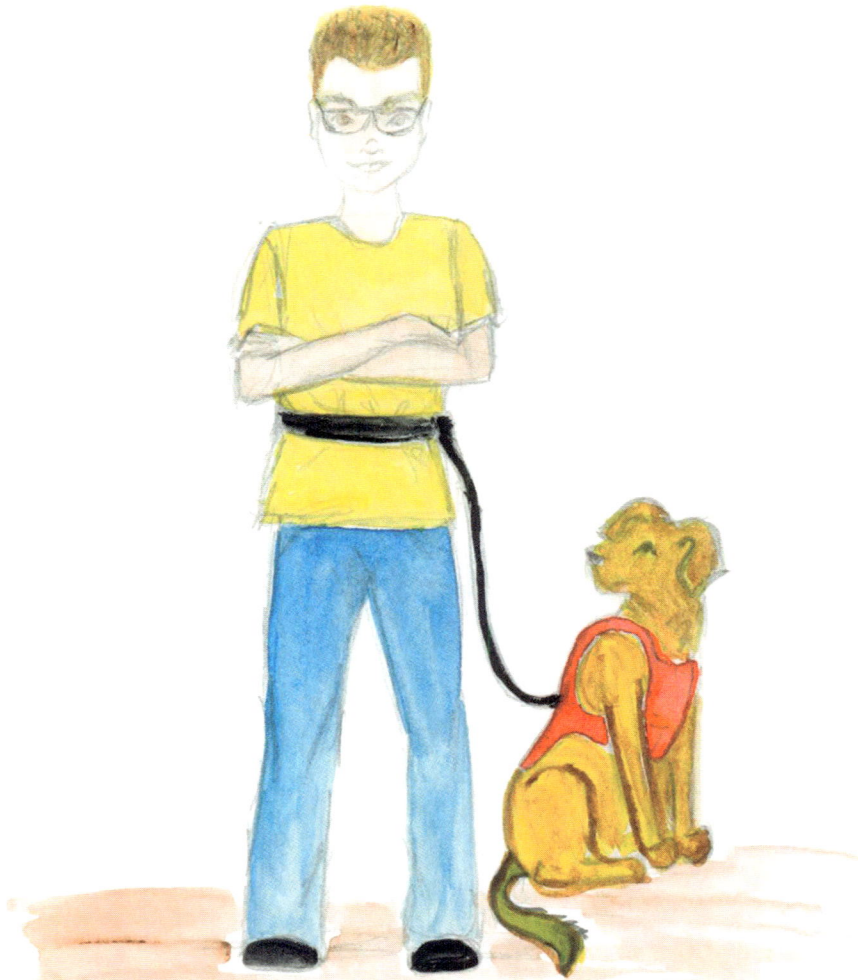

Ben was a 12-year-old boy with Autism. You couldn't see his disability until you spent some time talking to him. He was very good with numbers and could tell every highway exit across the state of Tennessee, but he needed someone with him all the time to keep him safe. It was hard for him not to wander off and get into trouble. Annie would be tethered to Ben and she would walk with him and keep him where he needed to be. She could also tell if Ben was ready to have what his mother called a "meltdown." She could bring him down to the floor and comfort him so that he could calm down. Sometimes Ben would become agitated when he had to do things too quickly. He liked to do things a certain way and when he couldn't he would be very upset. He didn't really know why, and it didn't seem like a good reason to be angry after it was over, but he simply could not stop it, until he started working with Annie. She was his best friend.

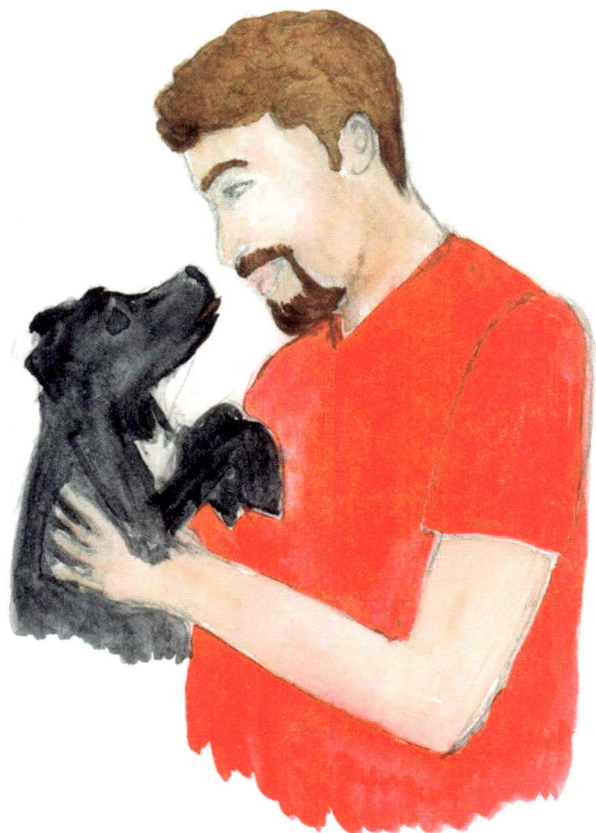

Matt was a 42-year-old man who had been wounded in the Army. You would not think that Matt was wounded by looking at him. He seemed like a regular guy. The doctors said that he had Post Traumatic Stress Disorder. Some days it was hard for Matt to get out of bed. After working with Manny, Matt looked forward to meeting Nicole for an outing with his new friend. Manny helped Matt when he was feeling anxious. Manny would lean on Matt and before long Matt would relax and lean on Manny and Manny would know that Matt was calm.

Bill told some of his coworkers about Ella and her puppies. The news traveled and someone decided that since Ella had chosen to come to Dollywood, they wanted to bring her back with all of her puppies and their families. Emily received a letter in the mail from Dollywood and enclosed were passes for everyone. Emily called Wilderwood and all the foster families as well as each of the new owners. She called Sadie and told her the news. Sadie was thrilled and asked Emily to send her pictures of the fun.

They all showed up and gathered excitedly at the front entrance. The first thing they did was go to get handicapped passes for the rides. They checked the show lists and decided which shows they might want to see if there was time. They discussed what rides everyone wanted to go on while they were there. They gathered at the train for a group photo and a FaceTime chat with Sadie. She was in tears as she saw their faces. It was like a dream come true for so many. The whole gang boarded the train and took a ride through the park. They were like one big happy family; so happy because of Ella. She was one very special dog!

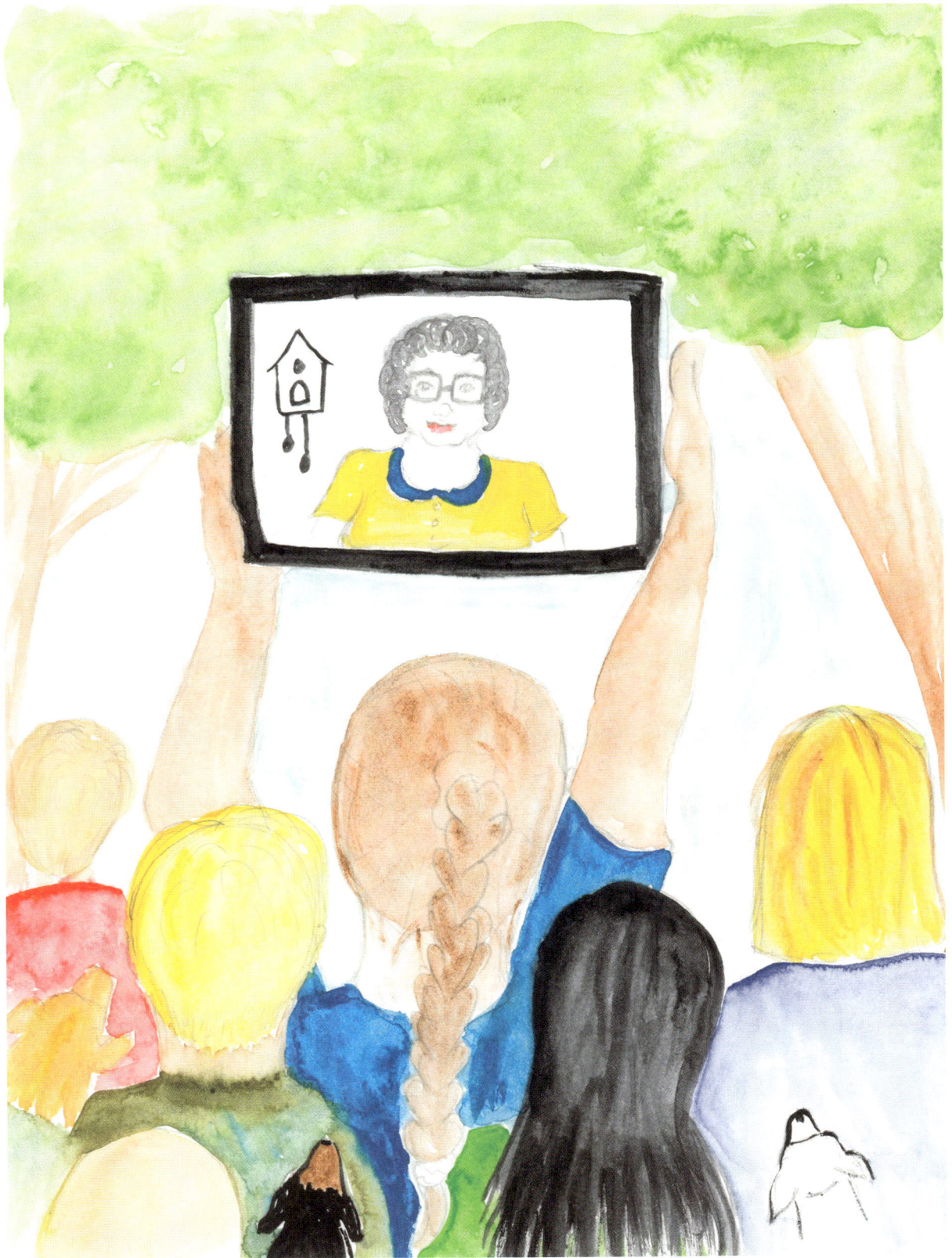

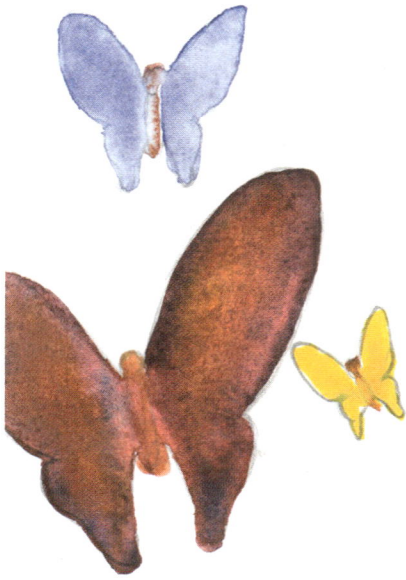
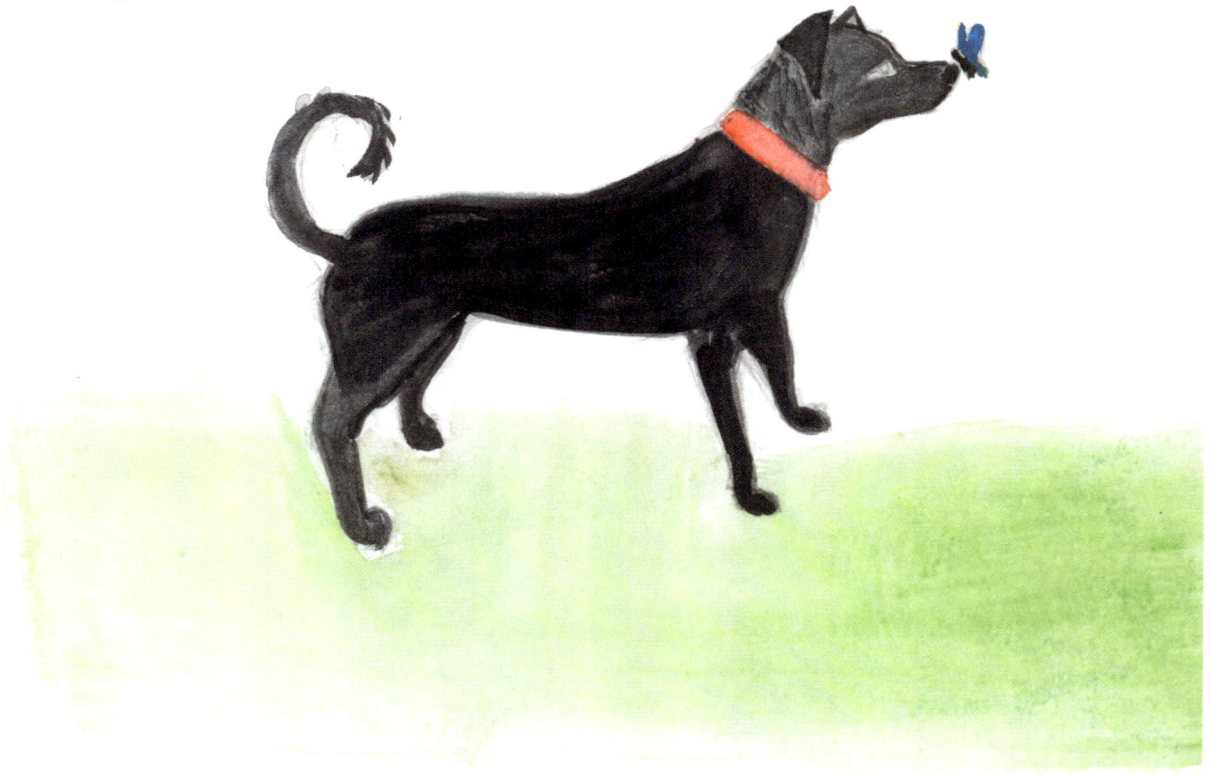

WILDERWOOD

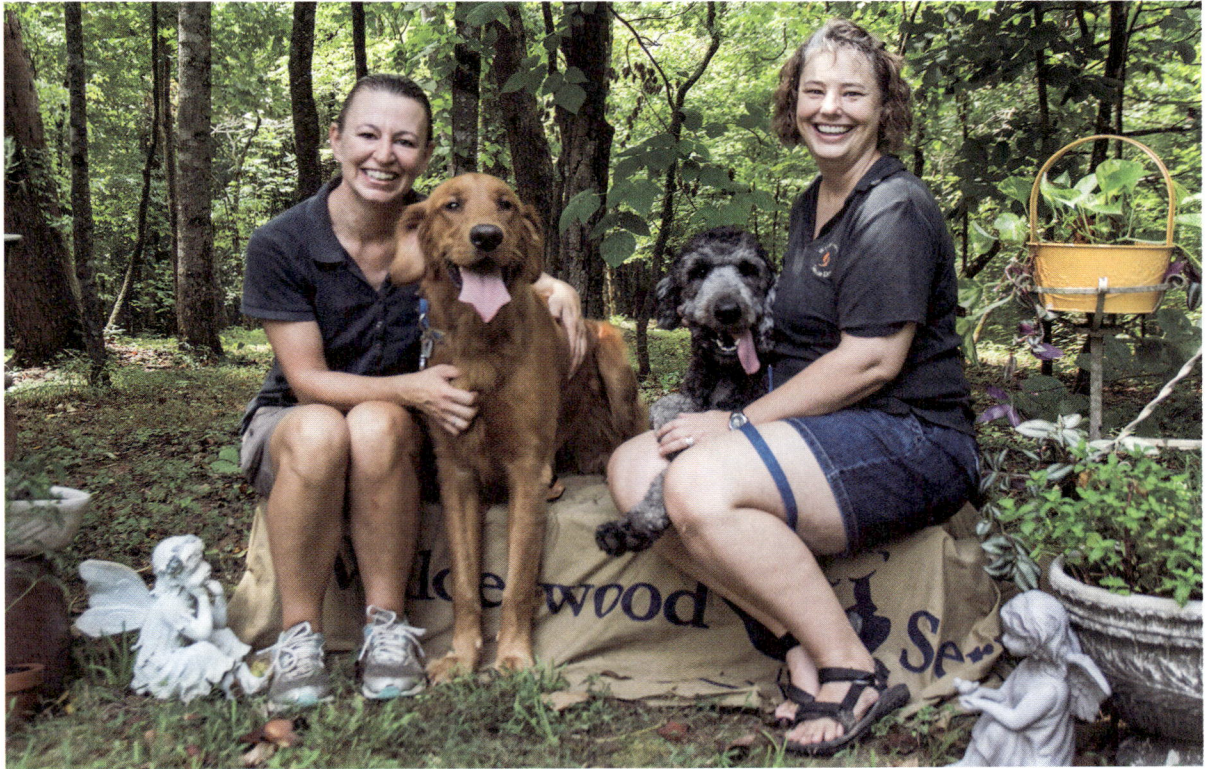

Nichole and Tiffany

Hello, my name is Tiffany and I'm the president/founder of Wilderwood. This organization was born out of dreams, sweat and tears, and I'm proud to be a part of it. We opened our doors in Maryville, Tennessee on August 1, 2005. I am a psychiatric nurse by degree and have been involved in psych care and nursing for most of my adult life. I have seen a lot of treatment modalities in that time. I have given a lot of medication. I deal daily with brain trauma, autism, emotional illness, dementia, and Alzheimer's. Out of these experiences arose an awareness that there was something missing and something that simply MUST work better.

I have also been involved with dogs since childhood. I have trained dogs in obedience, animal assisted therapy and service dog work. Wilderwood is an outgrowth of those life experiences.

In all my experience, I have never seen anything, and I can safely say ANYTHING, that has been more therapeutic than the animal/human interaction. What happens to a person's soul, and then their perception, in the presence of a beloved animal is far reaching. That relationship impacts a person's life more than a therapist, medicine, treatment programs or all of them combined. In that reality, Wilderwood finds its passion. Our dogs help individuals gain independence (emotional and physical). Our dogs provide unconditional love and support. They assist in all facets of life; behavioral, emotional and physical. I am excited to be a part of something so wonderful.

I have been working with Tiffany and Wilderwood Service Dogs for three years. It has been the most wonderful thing that I have ever had the honor of being a part of. Not only do I work with awesome dogs and fantastic fosters but I have met real life superheroes. Some of the strongest people I know are those with disabilities. I think the most amazing are the mothers of our Autistic kids. It is such a blessing to be a part of their journey with their service dog.   Nichole Ballard

Let's Go To The Arc

We can paint and we can sing; we enjoy our favorite things at The Arc.

We can clean and we're a team; we can laugh and we can dream at The Arc.

Oh, Oh, Let's go to The Arc

We can make a thank you card; we can help when life gets hard at The Arc.

We can draw and we can cook; we can read library books at The Arc.

Oh, Oh, Let's go to The Arc

We have many volunteers who stay friends throughout the years at The Arc.

We have parents who support and are always in our court at The Arc.

Oh, Oh, Let's go to The Arc

Let's go to The Arc

Let's go to The Arc

Let's go to The Arc

Let's go to The Arc

Oh, Oh, Let's go to The Arc

Oh, Oh, Let's go to The Arc

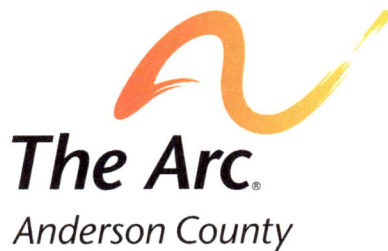

The Arc.
Anderson County

Our mission - to promote advocacy, empowerment, and full participation for people with intellectual and/or developmental disabilities

Our vision - to be a community that recognizes and embraces people in all abilities

Our Core Values - Teamwork, Helpfulness, Experience, Acceptance, Resourcefulness, Capability

The Arc Anderson County is a chapter of **The Arc of Tennessee** and **The Arc US**. Every chapter is different in that they speak to the needs in their community. The Arc Anderson County created an After School Program and a Summer program for participants to have a safe place to come together to learn, create and gain confidence. We have witnessed success in big ways and small ways. We realized how appropriate our program name was as our friends graduated from High School, then different programs, and came back to us part time. They still needed us in their lives.

We do short plays each year at our annual Dove Awards, dinner and a show, we have written our own song, and now this book. Who knows where life will take us, as long as our hearts and minds are open to new and different options? We hope you will follow us in our journey. Thank you for believing in our abilities.

Dargie Arwood, the Executive Director created The Arc AC After School and Summer Programs originally with volunteers. She works tirelessly with and for the I/DD Population in Oak Ridge, Tennessee and the surrounding area.

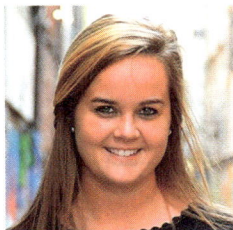

Jenna Murphy is our assistant teacher in our Arc AC, After School Program. She models our core values for our students. She restores our faith in the next generation. We know that Jenna will succeed in all that she attempts. We value her creativeness, kindness and patience as we all learn together.

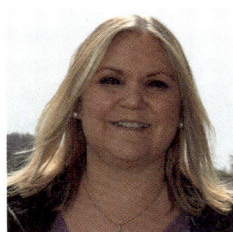

Beverly Joyce came to us when we were in desperate need, looking for a volunteer position for her daughter. She settled in as our lead teacher after 2 weeks of volunteering. We are thankful for her presence for the past 2 years. She has expanded our world with music, plays, books, and organization. She has a way of encouraging the students, pushing and expecting, to rise to higher heights than they thought possible. We are thankful for her guidance and willingness to be a part of our team.

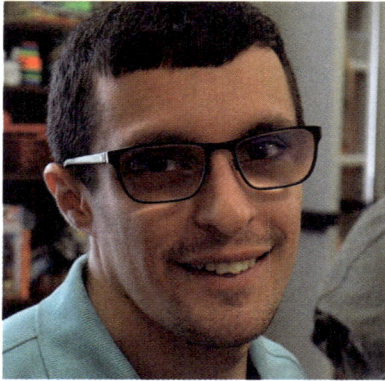

Alex has been a part of The Arc ASP since we started 4 years ago. He completed the UT Futures Program and has a job now but he still comes back to see us. Alex loves telephones from all eras, writing notes of encouragement, and spending time with friends. We could totally see him having his own office one day soon. He entertains us with feats of strength and funny voices.

Alexis A is homeschooled and travels almost an hour to The Arc AC. She loves art, science projects and spending time with friends. She has been in several plays and is always exploring amazing places, opportunities, and events. Thankfully she comes and shares her experiences with us.

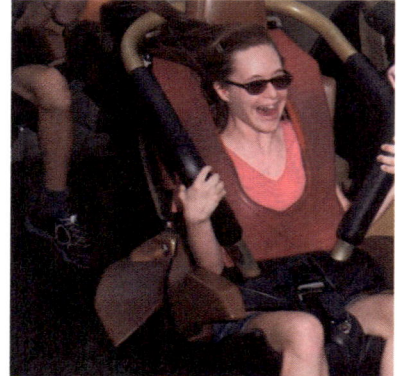

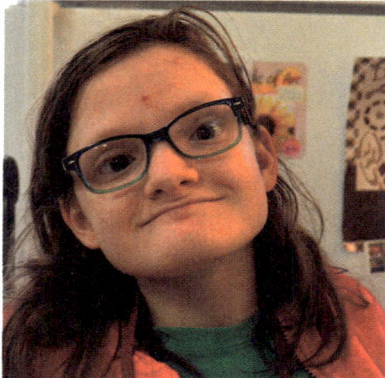

Alexis B rolled right into our hearts in her pink wheelchair with lights on its wheels. She is a soft spoken and kind young lady that is always willing to assist her friends. She loves keeping her hands busy with anything creative, but doesn't like loud noises. She is amazingly self sufficient and we are blessed to have her in our program.

Andrew is curious and full of laughter. He loves roller coasters and hanging out with friends. If there is a job to be done, Andrew is always willing to help us out. He is amazing on computers. He can go places that others might never know exist. He also knows every song we can think of.

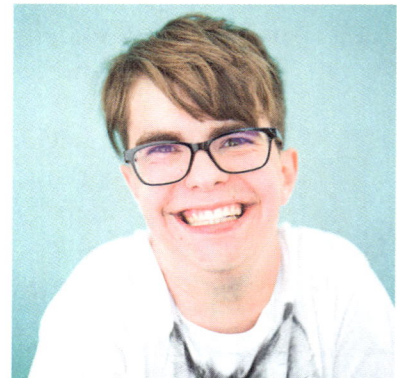

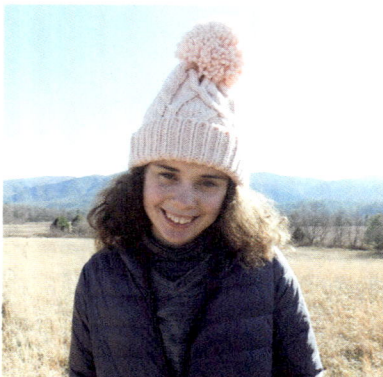

Autumn is an amazing young lady. She is such an important part of her family and our program because she consistently shows kindness and inclusion to everyone. She loves doing puzzles and is always willing to help others learn to do them as well. If a new person enters our classroom, they always have a friend if Autumn is there.

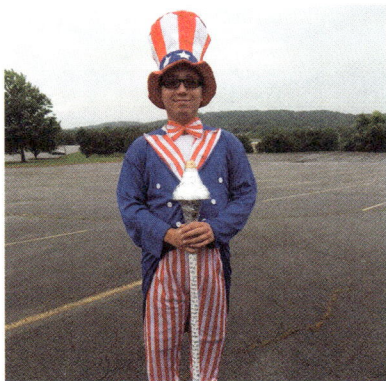

D'Andre is maturing into a fine man. We miss him so because he completed a local program and was able to get a wonderful job. He visits, but we miss his smiling face, encouraging words and his eagerness to help with anything we needed him to do. D'Andre is definitely going places, reaching higher heights and we wish him all the best.

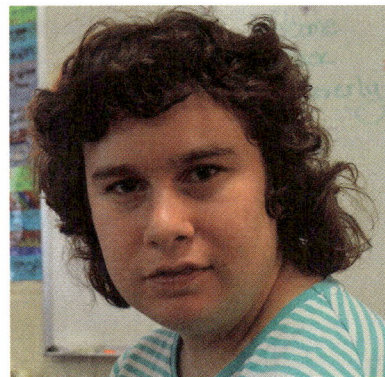

Erika is a pleasure to have in our program. She has a wonderful voice and a sincere servant's heart. She can handle any gadget we present to her and operate it with confidence. She is very sweet and kind and always makes us smile. She loves doing unique creations with arts and crafts.

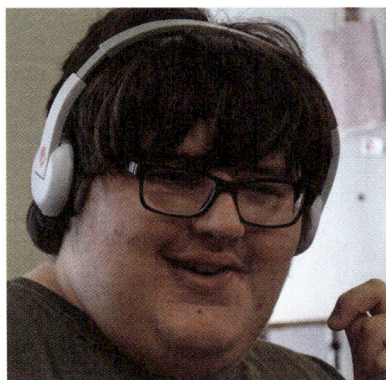

Ethan joined us recently at The Arc AC. He is always willing to help out. He makes us laugh and we have to remind him to let others have a turn when solving puzzles because he is so good at it. He is quite the artist and loves music. We look forward to him playing the cowardly lion in our performance of "The Wizard of OZ" this May.

George is a sensitive guy. He loves his church, his friends and his family, especially his dog, Charlotte. (She was kind enough to pose as Ella.) George has been focusing on getting a place of his own and a job. He visits us now and then and he will always be a part of our Arc family.

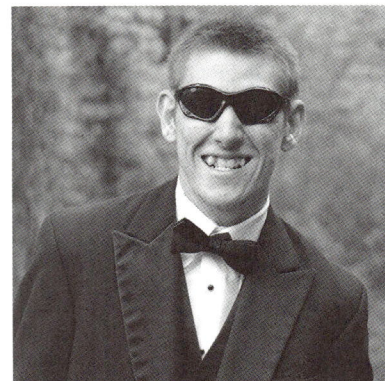

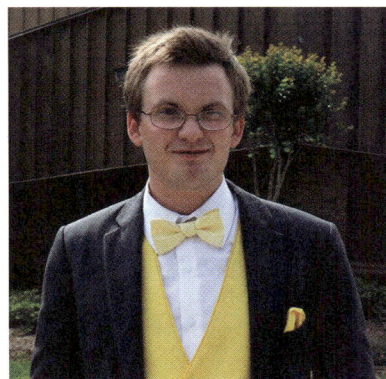

Joshua is a ray of sunshine. Perhaps that is the reason that his favorite color is yellow. He loves computers, game shows and numbers in general. Joshua astounds people with his knowledge of highway exits across Tennessee. Books and music are among his most prized possessions. Joshua did not start talking until a bit later than most, but we all soon realized that he has always had a lot to say. All we really have to do is listen.

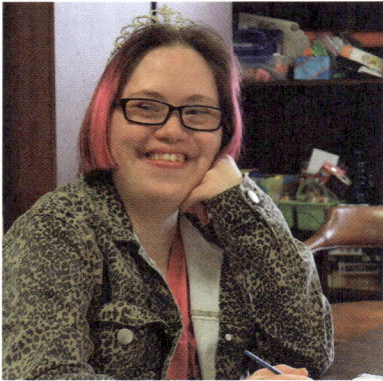

Katy is a young lady that loves cats, pink hair and tiaras. She sports attire that coincides with the holidays often with matching head gear. This girl can spin a basketball on her finger and makes more baskets than not when we play basketball. She loves to perform, is devoted to her friends and adores painting. Katy writes us wonderful notes and has quite a sense of humor. She remembers birthdays and how old people are like nobody I know.

Mark comes part time to The Arc AC. He is happy most of the time, and loves music-any kind of music. Mark does not speak, so we all have to work together to understand his language. He is a great addition to our group because he pushes others to understand things and look at life in a different way.

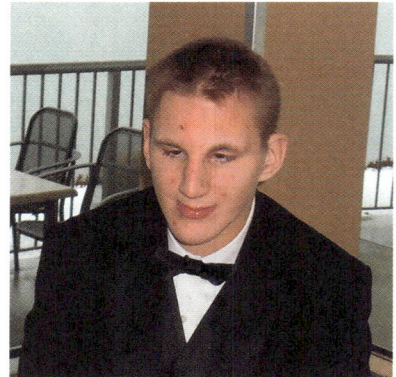

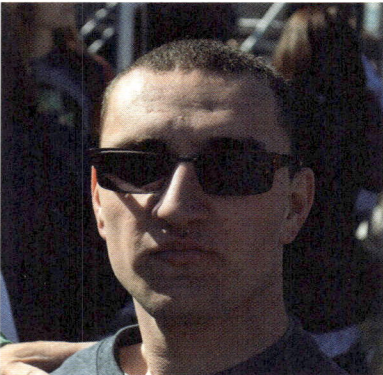

Zachary is sports oriented to the max! We love his enthusiasm. Zachary is kind and always happy to see his friends and even more so if there is a competition involved. Zachary is great with details and always willing to learn and try new things.